BACK SCHOOL
AND OTHER CONSERVATIVE
APPROACHES TO LOW BACK PAIN

MOSBY   YEAR BOOK

TIMES MIRROR

WITH COMPLIMENTS FROM
ROGER TOMLINSON

Barnard's Inn, Holborn, London EC1N 2JA. ENGLAND.
Telephone No: 01-242 9613   Telex No: 268633

BACK SCHOOL AND OTHER CONSERVATIVE APPROACHES TO LOW BACK PAIN

ARTHUR H. WHITE, M.D.

Director, St. Mary's Spine Center; Founder,
California Back School; and Senior Spine Consultant,
San Francisco Orthopaedic Residency Program,
San Francisco, California

Collaborators

Lynne A. White

Health Education Systems, Inc.,
Tiburon, California

A. William Mattmiller, R.P.T.

Physical Therapy Consultant and
Director, San Francisco Back School,
St. Mary's Hospital Spine Center,
San Francisco, California

with **83** illustrations

The C. V. Mosby Company

ST. LOUIS • TORONTO • LONDON   **1983**

MOSBY

A TRADITION OF PUBLISHING EXCELLENCE

Editor: Eugenia Klein
Developmental editor: Kathy Falk
Manuscript editor: Selena V. Bussen
Book design: Kay M. Kramer
Cover design: Diane Beasley
Production: Linda R. Stalnaker, Barbara Merritt

The C.V. Mosby Company
11830 Westline Industrial Drive, St. Louis, Missouri 63141

Library of Congress Cataloging in Publication Data

White, Arthur H., 1938-
    Back school and other conservative approaches
to low back pain.

    Bibliography: p.
    Includes index.
    1. Backache—Treatment. I. Title. [DNLM:
1. Backache—Therapy. WE 755 W582b]
RD768.W429 1982   617'.56   82-12541
ISBN 0-8016-5423-8

AC/VH/VH   9 8 7 6 5 4 3 2 1   01/C/070

PREFACE

Education has been the major tool used by society to make advancements. Medicine has used education to help eradicate innumerable diseases such as the plague, tuberculosis, poliomyelitis, malaria, and typhoid fever.

As medical practitioners, in our daily war against illness on a one-to-one basis, we are so busy treating the patients at hand that we frequently forget about the tool of education. We are taught to treat, not to teach.

Now that medicine has conquered many of the "more important" life-threatening diseases, attention has been turned toward the multi-billion-dollar bothersome back problem. Surgery, pills, manipulations, injections, and other conservative measures have not even been able to hold the low back problem constant. It is a rapidly growing social, medical, psychological, surgical, and industrial dilemma.

In our fight against low back pain, we must return to the weapon that we have experienced as working best in the past—education. Low back pain is preventable and controllable. We must educate ourselves and our patients as to the cause of low back pain, so that they can take responsibility in the prevention and control of their own conditions.

The back school is the center from which we can disseminate education to all of the segments of society who are responsible for or suffering from the low back dilemma.

It is hoped that this book will reawaken interest in educating patients to help them maintain an attitude of well-being and avoid the unnecessary abuses that we unknowingly impose on our bodies.

For the sake of clarity and simplicity, the male pronoun has been used to refer to the physician, therapist, and patient, even though we fully recognize the fact that there are women in this area of medicine. We certainly realize, too, that women, as well as men, suffer from low back pain.

I thank Harry Fahrni for being who I consider the father of back school. His 20 years of working with the principles of back school before 1970 provided the latticework on which we were able to build.

Innumerable therapists, nurses, physicians, and other associates provided the innovations and footwork that have allowed back school to become one of the fastest-growing subspecialties in medicine today. It is impossible to mention specifically all of these individuals who have helped the development of the back school concept. It was, however, my wife, Lynne, and Bill Mattmiller, who worked with me on a daily basis for the past 10 years, in developing and using all of the principles in this text. Chris Shulenberger has been a great asset in developing ergonomics in our back school model. David

Schmidt, Ellen Fineman, and Patty Vicas have been of invaluable assistance in training patients and demonstrating the principles of their work, as photographically illustrated by Rick Soloway.

I want to thank Eugenia Klein, Kathy Falk, and Jerri Holmes for their editorial and organizational assistance and their tolerance.

Special gratitude goes to my patients and students who teach me through our work together and who are actively disseminating this information to others.

Arthur H. White

CONTENTS

1   The etiology of low back pain and patient evaluation, 1

2   Classification of low back pain, 26

3   History of back school, 43

4   Basic back school, 48

5   Hospital back school, 82

6   Back school in the home environment, 107

7   Back school in the work environment, 141

8   Athletic back school, 157

9   Other conservative measures, 169

10   The future of back school, 177

References and suggested readings, 181

1 THE ETIOLOGY OF LOW BACK PAIN AND PATIENT EVALUATION

ETIOLOGY

For hundreds of years there has been a great mystery about the source of low back pain. Ancient demons were released by drilling holes in the head. The more modern demons have been cured by ultrasound waves, electrical stimuli, acupuncture, and medication. After the discovery of the significance of the herniated lumbar disc in the mid-1930s, there was a scientific explosion of experimental data about low back pain. Innumerable papers have been published on patients' complaints, predisposing factors for low back pain, various treatments and their successes, and every conceivable biomechanical and pathophysiological study. These scientific laboratory experiments have required modern laboratories that can measure intradiscal pressure, intraabdominal pressure, microscopic blood flow, autoimmune changes in the blood, chemical changes in the blood and urine, and the ultramicroscopic appearance of the lumbar structures. All of this has led to the modern concept of the cause of low back pain. Although we do not know all of the sources of low back pain, it is universally agreed that the degenerating lumbar segment produces significant physical changes in the facet joints, discs, and intervertebral structures that are associated with nerve endings. There are more scientific data to support the degenerating intervertebral segment, over any other structure, as the source of most low back pain.

The degenerating lumbar segment is basically an aging process. This aging process begins to become painful at approximately 35 years of age in the average individual in an industrialized society. In other, more primitive cultures, where people use their backs differently, such as the ground-dwelling populations, the degenerative segment does not become a painful clinical entity until much later in life. These ground-dwelling populations spend much of the time squatting and sitting on the ground with the distribution of forces on the intervertebral segment being much different from that in societies where people sit in chairs and spend most of their time in an erect posture. Excessive lumbar lordosis, obesity, pregnancy, weak abdominal muscles, and long periods of standing predispose persons in industrialized societies to excessive forces on the posterior aspects of the lumbar disc.

There are entire books written on the reason for selecting one area of the spine as the primary degenerating aspect. The first histological change that we see in most studies is that of the anulus tear of the disc. This can be produced in the laboratory with a flexion and rotation positioning with loading. Clinically, we see this entity frequently, as the

1

patient states that he felt or heard something tear in his back while he was bending forward to pick up something. Further details with regard to the diagnostic findings in such cases are presented later.

Since degenerative disc disease is a normal aging process, it should not be considered a disease at all. Every disc goes through a normal day's worth of aging each day. It has some minimal ability to repair some of the aging during periods of rest. At the end of a lifetime, most discs have accumulated enough aging to be considered deteriorated, degenerated, or simply worn out. If the process takes 50 to 70 years to run its course, it is not necessarily painful. If, however, the process occurs rapidly, there may be episodes of days to years of low back pain.

It is equally plausible that the facet joints are the first to be injured. They, too, can cause an inflammatory process that produces a specific clinical syndrome. The resultant injury and possible hypermobility of the segment can then lead to disc deterioration. Either or both of these can be responsible for straining the other supporting structures of the segment, such as the ligaments and muscles. The most painful entity is neurological compression, which can give a severe degree of pain and lead to total incapacity and surgery.

There are innumerable other etiologies for the occurrence of low back pain. There are over a hundred diagnoses for low back pain. These causes can generally be categorized as congenital, traumatic, infectious, metabolic, degenerative, and neoplastic. The causes can be broken down into many other subheadings and even carried to the specific activity that is responsible for the low back pain, such as pregnancy, lifting, bending, or driving. All evidence suggests, however, that the most common cause of low back pain is the degenerative lumbar segment. This book deals mainly with the degenerative lumbar segment and the clinical presentations therefrom. Other vague entities, such as strains, sprains, and myofascitis, have little evidence for their existence. They may occasionally be a source of low back pain, and studies should continue in an attempt to scientifically validate these diagnoses.

Because there are so many nonspinal sources of low back pain, it is wise to do a complete history and physical examination early in the course of the disease. If the practitioner attempting to diagnose and treat back pain is not qualified or competent in the general medical aspects of a total physical evaluation, he should seek the assistance of someone with broader general medical knowledge and experience. There is nothing that will more quickly curtail our success and the confidence of our patients than the misdiagnosis of low back pain that turns out to be a cancer or other serious organ system disease.

The history and physical examination is the mainstay of most medical diagnoses. Each organ system must be reviewed by a history and physical examination to eliminate it as a source of pain.

PATIENT HISTORY

The history for spinal pain can be quite extensive. It is sometimes helpful to have many of the routine questions asked by means of a questionnaire (Fig. 1-1). A nurse or therapist may ask additional questions. Other aids, such as the pain drawing, can save many words on the part of the patient and questions on the part of the physician. The most pertinent history to obtain in evaluating the degenerative segment is the mechanism of injury and the aggravating and relieving factors. Other less important, but nevertheless valuable, information includes the past occurrences of back pain along with the length of time they lasted, treatment, and responses to treatment. Underlying emotional factors, family histories, and compensation elements can also be important.

PATIENT HISTORY

Name_____ Age_____

Date_____ Date of injury_____

1. How long have you had the present pain?_____

2. Where is the pain located?_____

3. Do you have leg pain or leg cramping; if so, where?_____

    _____

4. Have you been hospitalized for your back pain?_____

    When?_____ How long?_____

5. If you were injured, how did your injury occur?_____

    Bending_____ Lifting_____ Twisting_____ Other_____

6. What type of work did (do) you do?_____

7. What specific pain or limitation keeps you from returning to normal

    function or work?_____

8. Are you able to care for yourself at home?_____ If not, what

    activities can't you do?_____

9. Are you doing normal housework?_____

10. How many hours in the day do you stand?_____

    Doing what?_____

11. How many hours in the day do you sit?_____

    Doing what?_____ What type of chair is most comfortable?_____

12. How many hours in the day do you drive or ride?_____

    What type of car?_____ What type of seat?_____

13. How many hours in the night do you sleep?_____

    In what position do you sleep?_____

    On what type of mattress?_____ How old is the mattress?_____

14. Do you do any lifting?_____ What kind?_____

    Weight?_____ How often?_____

15. What treatments, if any, have made your pain better?_____

16. What treatments, if any, have made your pain worse?_____

17. How long can you sit comfortably?_____

18. How long can you stand comfortably?_____

19. How far can you walk comfortably?_____

Continued.

Fig. 1-1. Patient history.

```
20.  Please check if your pain is better, worse, or unchanged with the_____
     following activities:
                                              Better    Worse    Unchanged
     Coughing or sneezing                     _____    _____   _____
     Sitting down at a table                  _____    _____   _____
     Sitting in an automobile                 _____    _____   _____

     Bending forward to brush my teeth        _____    _____   _____
     Walking a short distance                 _____    _____   _____
     Lying flat on my back                    _____    _____   _____
     Lying on my side with knees bent         _____    _____   _____

     When I awaken in the morning             _____    _____   _____
     Middle of the night                      _____    _____   _____
     Mid-day                                  _____    _____   _____

     Reaching                                 _____    _____   _____
     Squatting                                _____    _____   _____
     Twisting                                 _____    _____   _____
     Pushing a vacuum or grocery cart         _____    _____   _____

21.  What do you do for recreation or sports?_____

22.  What would you like to do?_____

23.  To what type of work, if any, do you anticipate returning?_____

24.  Has your doctor explained to you what is wrong with your back?_____

25.  What are your goals for your back problem?_____
```

Fig. 1-1, cont'd. Patient history.

A good method of taking a current pain history is to ask patients to describe a typical 24-hour period. They list the activities performed and the type, location, and severity of pain. For example, how many times do they awaken at night with pain? How do they feel when they first wake up in the morning, when they get out of bed, when they brush their teeth, and when they sit down for breakfast?

Because emotional factors are frequently involved with low back pain, psychological testing may be indicated. We need to delve into the patient's feelings about his condition and the interference in his normal life patterns. It is important to know whether he has an attorney and what secondary gains are involved. This could play a part psychologically.

Many physicians feel that they can look at a patient and tell whether he is "nuts." Many of us feel we are good judges of character and can spot a phony or a gold-bricker a mile away. Obviously the medical profession is not doing a very good job in this identification. This is verified by the thousands of individuals in pain clinics who have had many operations and continue to have back pain. In retrospect we state that the pain was all on a psychological or emotional basis to begin with. It is not reasonable to make a premature diagnosis on an emotional patient and then fail to relieve the pain with surgery and say, "Oh well, this patient is nuts anyway." We need to identify and treat the patient's psychological problems as well as the objective physical pathology. Listening to the patient is one of the most important ways of identifying the many contributing factors in each case. In our busy practices we do not take time to listen to the patient long enough to determine that there are many factors in addition to the physical diagnosis.

We use a functional rating scale (boxed material on p. 5) in our clinic, giving points for inconsistencies in the patient's history and physical evaluation, the presence of important industrial factors, the presence of an attorney in the case, psychological testing, and

Functional rating

NAME:
DATE:
DIAGNOSIS:
AGE:

Points	Explanation
1	Industrial
1	Inconsistent history (allergies, headaches, no relief with rest, accompanied by mate)
1	Inconsistent examination (burns, flip, dramatic, and unrealistic)
1	Pain threshold
1	Surveillance
1	Legal
1	Pain drawing
3	MMPI (Hs or Hy greater than 70)

---

pain threshold. If the patient accumulates more than two points on such a scale, he is suspected of having significant emotional contribution to the low back pain.

Other objective tests are available that are useful not only in helping the physician evaluate the patient with low back pain, but in helping the patient develop stressor identification skills. These tests include the Social Readjustment Rating Scale (SRRS), the Hendler 10-Minute Screening Test for Chronic Back Pain, and the Personal Concerns Inventory.

FUNCTIONAL RATING SCALE

Each patient is to receive a functional rating on the basis of points from 1 to 10 (box above). Each medical and paramedical individual who is associated with the patient circles the number in the point column that he has identified as being abnormal. For instance, the secretary can identify the industrial and legal aspects and perhaps participate in the surveillance. The therapist sees the inconsistent history and the pain drawing and identifies the low pain threshold and any inconsistency on examination. When the Minnesota Multiphasic Personality Inventory (MMPI) is done, whoever grades it will circle the appropriate points. Open observation of the obstacle course, exercise performance, and positioning throughout all back school activities, and when necessary, clandestine observation of the patient in the hallway is done as surveillance.

Add points in this manner:

1 Work related or industrial accident.

1 Inconsistent history, inconsistent findings, unconfirmed or vague diagnosis.

1 An invalid, manipulated or dramatic presentation, or physical evaluation.

1 A pain scale rating above 4 on either the pain drawing or reported during activity, especially the wall sit time.

1   An obvious manipulation of symptoms, demonstrative activity, inconsistent use of body mechanics, or lack of cooperation.

1   A legal case or a lawyer is involved.

1   A pain drawing demonstrating diffuse, nonanatomical, extrasomatic, or unrealistic pains for that diagnosis.

1   Every score (Hs and Hy) above 70% on the MMPI.

SOCIAL READJUSTMENT RATING SCALE

The Social Readjustment Rating Scale (Fig. 1-2) evaluates events that correlate with levels of emotional stress by assigning a point value to these events. For example, the recent death of a spouse is worth 100 points, a son or daughter leaving home is worth 29 points, and a change in social activities is worth 18 points.

Forty-three questions are included on the SRRS. These questions may be asked during a clinical examination and scored in a minimum of time. In clinical practice scores between 30 and 200 are normal. Scores over 200 may indicate patients who are likely to have a significant emotional component to their low back pain.

SOCIAL READJUSTMENT RATING SCALE

Rank	Life event	Mean value
1	Death of spouse	100
2	Divorce	73
3	Marital separation	65
4	Jail term	63
5	Death of close family member	63
6	Personal injury or illness	53
7	Marriage	50
8	Fired at work	47
9	Marital reconciliation	45
10	Retirement	45
11	Change in health of family member	44
12	Pregnancy	40
13	Sex difficulties	39
14	Gain of new family member	39
15	Business readjustment	39
16	Change in financial state	38
17	Death of close friend	37
18	Change to different line of work	36
19	Change in number of arguments with spouse	35
20	Mortgage over $10,000	31
21	Foreclosure of mortgage or loan	30
22	Change in responsibilities at work	29
23	Son or daughter leaving home	29
24	Trouble with in-laws	29
25	Outstanding personal achievement	28
26	Wife beginning or stopping work	26
27	Beginning or ending school	26
28	Change in living conditions	25
29	Revision of personal habits	24
30	Trouble with boss	23
31	Change in work hours or conditions	20
32	Change in residence	20
33	Change in schools	20
34	Change in recreation	19
35	Change in church activities	19
36	Change in social activities	18
37	Mortgage or loan less than $10,000	17
38	Change in sleeping habits	16
39	Change in number of family get-togethers	15
40	Change in eating habits	15
41	Vacation	13
42	Christmas	12
43	Minor violations of the law	11

Fig. 1-2. Social readjustment rating scale.
Adapted from Holmes, T.H., and Rahe, R.H.: The social readjustment rating scale, J. Psychosom. Res. **11**:213-218, 1967.

HENDLER 10-MINUTE SCREENING TEST FOR CHRONIC BACK PAIN PATIENTS

The Hendler 10-Minute Screening Test (Fig. 1-3) is merely a screening procedure and not a diagnostic tool, and clinical judgment must be exercised at all times.

Although the test was originally designed to evaluate the emotional components that may effect the verbalization of chronic pain, it has been used successfully in evaluating patients with low back pain. In fact it was designed specifically for low back pain as well as neck, arm, shoulder, and leg pain. However, it is not applicable for headache, chest pain, or abdominal pain. It differentiates between patients with a normal or typical response to painful conditions, patients who are likely to be exaggerating their complaints, and patients who may have serious psychiatric illness.

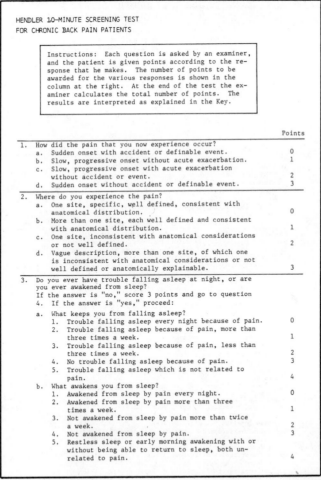

Continued.

Fig. 1-3. Hendler 10-minute screening test for chronic back pain patients.

Adapted from Hendler, N., et al.: A preoperative screening test for chronic back pain patients, Psychosomatics **20** (12): 801-808, Dec. 1979. This test may not be reproduced without expressed permission at Nelson Hendler, M.D., Clinical Director, Mensana Clinic, Greenspring Valley Rd., Stevenson, Md. 21153.

	Points
4. Does weather have any effect on your pain?	
a. The pain is always worse in both cold *and* damp weather.	0
b. The pain is always worse in cold weather *or* in damp weather.	1
c. The pain is occasionally worse in cold or damp weather.	2
d. The weather has no effect on the pain.	3
5. How would you describe the type of pain that you have?	
a. Burning, or sharp, shooting pain, or pins and needles, or coldness, or numbness.	0
b. Dull, aching pain, with occasional sharp, shooting pains not helped by heat, or hyperesthesia.	1
c. Spasm-type pain, tension-type pain, or numbness over the area relieved by massage or heat.	2
d. Nagging or bothersome pain.	3
e. Excruciating, overwhelming, or unbearable pain relieved by massage or heat.	4
6. How frequently do you have your pain?	
a. The pain is constant.	0
b. The pain is nearly constant, occurring 50% to 80% of the time.	1
c. The pain is intermittent, occurring 25% to 50% of the time.	2
d. The pain is only occasionally present, occurring less than 25% of the time.	3
7. Does movement or position have any effect on the pain?	
a. The pain is unrelieved by position change or rest, and there have been previous operations for the pain.	0
b. The pain is worsened by use, standing, or walking, and is relieved by lying down or resting.	1
c. Position change and use have variable effects on the pain.	2
d. The pain is not altered by use or position change, and there have been no previous operations for the pain.	3
8. What medications have you used in the past month?	
a. No medications at all.	0
b. Use of non-narcotic pain relievers, nonbenzodiazepine tranquilizers, or antidepressants.	1
c. Use of a narcotic, hypnotic, or benzodiazepine less than three times a week.	2
d. Use of a narcotic, hypnotic, or benzodiazepine more than four times a week.	3
9. What hobbies do you have, and can you still participate in them?	
a. Unable to participate in any hobbies that were formerly enjoyed.	0
b. Reduced number of hobbies or activities relating to a hobby.	1
c. Still able to participate in hobbies but with some discomfort.	2
d. Able to participate in hobbies as before.	3
10. How frequently did you have sex and orgasms before the pain, and how frequently do you have sex and orgasms now?	
a. 1. Prior to pain, sexual contact three to four times a week with no difficulty with orgasm; now frequency of sexual contact is 50% or less, and coitus is interrupted by pain.	0
2. (For people over 45) Sexual contact twice a week with a 50% reduction in frequency since the onset of pain.	0
3. (For people over 60) Sexual contact once a week with a 50% reduction in frequency since the onset of pain.	0
b. Sexual adjustment before pain as defined above with no difficulty with orgasm; now loss of interest in sex and/or difficulty with orgasm or erection.	1
c. No change in sexual activity.	2
d. Unable to have sexual contact since the onset of pain and difficulty with orgasm or erection *prior to* the pain.	3
e. No sexual contact prior to the pain or absence of orgasm *prior to* the pain.	4
11. Are you still working or doing your household chores?	
a. Works every day at the same job before pain or same level of household duties.	0
b. Works every day, but the job, with reduced responsibility or physical activity, is not the same as job before pain.	1
c. Works sporadically or does a reduced amount of household chores.	2
d. Not working or all household chores are now performed by others.	3

Fig. 1-3, cont'd. Hendler 10-minute screening test for chronic back pain patients.

	Points
12. What is your income now, compared with before your injury or the onset of pain, and what are your sources of income?	
a. Any one of the following answers scores	0
1. Experiencing financial difficulty, with family income 50% or less than previously.	
2. Retired.	
3. Still working and not having financial difficulty.	
b. Experiencing financial difficulty, with family income only 50% to 75% of the income before pain.	1
c. Unable to work and receives some compensation so that the family income is at least 75% of the income before pain.	2
d. Unable to work and receives no compensation, but the spouse works and family income is still 75% of the income before pain.	3
e. Not working, yet the income from disability or other compensation sources is 80% or more of gross pay before the pain; the spouse does not work.	4
13. Are you suing anyone, or is anyone suing you, or do you have an attorney helping you with compensation or disability payments?	
a. No suit pending and does not have an attorney.	0
b. Litigation is pending but is not related to the pain.	1
c. Being sued as the result of an accident.	2
d. Litigation is pending or workmen's compensation case with a lawyer involved.	3
14. If you had three wishes for anything in the world, what would you wish for?	
a. "Get rid of the pain" is the only wish.	0
b. "Get rid of the pain" is one of the three wishes.	1
c. Does not mention getting rid of the pain, but has specific wishes, usually of a personal nature, such as for more money, a better relationship with spouse or children, etc.	2
d. Does not mention pain but offers general, nonpersonal wishes, such as for world peace.	3
15. Have you ever been depressed or thought of suicide?	
a. Admits to depression or has a history of depression secondary to pain and associated with crying spells and thoughts of suicide.	0
b. Admits to depression, guilt, and anger secondary to the pain.	1
c. Prior history of depression before the pain or a financial or personal loss prior to the pain; now admits to some depression.	2
d. Denies depression, crying spells, or "feeling blue."	3
e. History of a suicide attempt prior to the onset of pain.	4
POINT TOTAL	

KEY TO HENDLER SCREENING TEST
FOR CHRONIC BACK PAIN

A score of 18 points or less suggests that the patient is an objective pain patient and is reporting a normal response to chronic pain. One may proceed surgically if indicated. The patient usually is quite willing to participate in all modalities of therapy, including exercise and psychotherapy. Occasionally, a person with conversion reaction or neurosis following trauma will score less than 18 points. This is because subjective distress is being experienced on an unconscious level. Persons scoring 14 points or less can be considered objective pain patients with more certainty than those at the upper range (14 to 18) of this group.

A score of 15 to 20 points suggests that the patient has features of an objective pain patient as well as of an exaggerating pain patient. This implies that a person with a poor premorbid adjustment has an organic lesion that has produced the normal response to pain. However, because of the person's poor adjustment before pain, the chronic pain produces a more extreme response than would otherwise occur.

A score of 19 to 31 points suggests that the patient is an exaggerating pain patient. Surgical or other interventions may be carried out with caution. This type of patient usually has a premorbid (before pain) personality that may increase his likelihood of using or benefiting from the complaint of chronic pain. The patient may show improvement after treatment in a chronic pain treatment center where the main emphasis is placed on an attitude change toward the chronic pain.

A score of 32 points or more suggests that a psychiatric consultation is needed. These patients freely admit to a great many problems before pain and show considerable difficulty in coping with the chronic pain they now experience. Surgical or other interventions should not be carried out without prior approval of a psychiatric consultant. Severe depression, suicide, and psychosis are potential problems in this group of affective pain patients.

Test copyright 1979 by Nelson Hendler, M.D., M.S.

Fig. 1-3, cont'd. Hendler 10-minute screening test for chronic back pain patients.

PERSONAL CONCERNS INVENTORY

The Personal Concerns Inventory (PCI) (Fig. 1-4) is a patient self-assessment method. The PCI approach is for the patient to take numerical self-ratings of his own psychological disposition and of stress- and tension-related variables over a period of time. The total PCI score should decrease over time with the use of psychological consultations and relaxation therapy.

PERSONAL CONCERNS

A Program

DATE ______________

SEX ______ AGE ______ HEIGHT ______ WEIGHT ______

MARITAL STATUS ______________

	DAY 1	DAY 2	DAY 3	DAY 4	DAY 5	DAY 6	DAY 7	TOTAL	DAY 1	DAY 2
Need More Recreation										
Noise At Home										
Noise At Work										
Sleeping Problems										
Chest Pain										
Problems With Children										
Weight Problem										
Need to be More Assertive										
Recent Death in Family										
High Blood Pressure										
Conflicts With Relatives										
Poor Eating Habits										
Short Temper										
Freeway Traffic										
Cigarette Smoking										
Feel Guilty										
Back Pain										
Alcohol (self)										
Alcohol (other)										
Jealousy										
Pill Consumption										
Boredom										
Tension										
Worry Too Much										
Medical Bills										
Need Employment										
Divorce										
Separation										
Dislike Job										
Continued Physical Pain										
Job Security										
Unexpressed Anger										
Headaches										
Trouble Making Decisions										
Conflicts With Neighbors										
Marital Problems										
Financial Difficulties										
Desire More Social Life										
Need to Relax										
Trouble With Employer										
Need Physical Exercise										
Need Friends										
Nervousness										
Sex Difficulties										
More Time for Myself										
Deadlines on Job										
Depression										
Can't Say No										
Ulcers										
Loneliness										
General Unhappiness										
More Self-discipline										
TOTAL										

Fig. 1-4. Personal concerns inventory.
Adapted from Mulry, R.C.: Personal concerns inventory. The back school: an audiovisual team approach to low back pain, St. Louis, 1981, The C.V. Mosby Co.

The patient is asked to rate each of 52 items every day for 21 days. Using the scale on the PCI, the patient is to consider each issue and indicate to what degree that issue is a concern to him on a day to day basis.

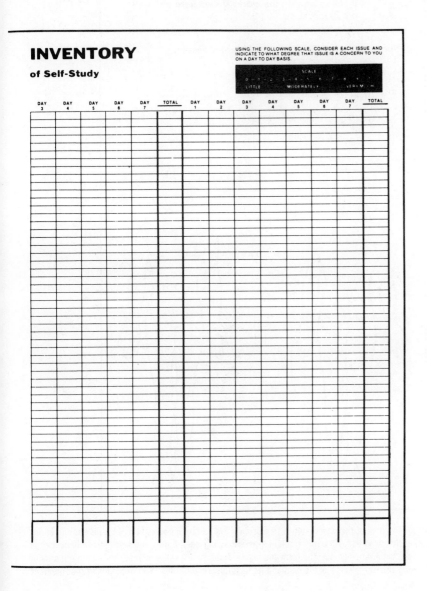

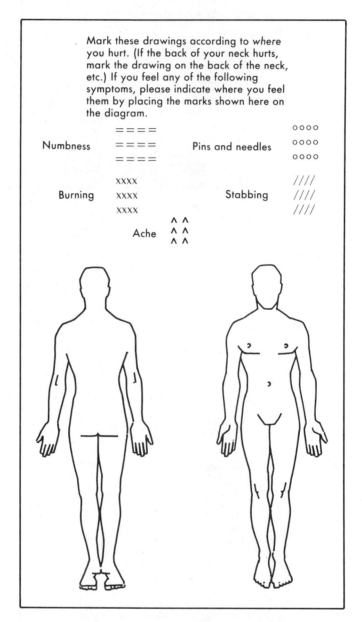

Mark these drawings according to *where* you hurt. (If the back of your neck hurts, mark the drawing on the back of the neck, etc.) If you feel any of the following symptoms, please indicate where you feel them by placing the marks shown here on the diagram.

Numbness   ====   Pins and needles   oooo

Burning   xxxx   Stabbing   ////

Ache   ^ ^

Fig. 1-5. Pain drawing. The goal of the pain drawn is to elucidate the patient's perception of his pain and to serve as a measuring device for progress. All patients fill in a pain drawing on the first and last days of back school whether or not they are experiencing pain. The form and legend symbols are self-explanatory. The patient should indicate on the drawing the percentage of his pain and its location and what his level of pain is at that moment while he is standing.

PAIN DRAWING

A pain drawing (Fig. 1-5) helps the physician determine a patient's perception of his pain. It indicates his personal involvement with the painful syndrome. A patient who is unusually preoccupied with his pain may make a drawing that is very dramatic and unrealistic. He tends to have drawings that are nonanatomical, or that pass outside of the drawing and even of the paper. Some of these patients create elaborate color schemes and make their own pain scales. Some patients will attempt to show the physician how bad they are with additional painful areas in the head, neck, and arms. The less emotionally involved patient makes a more careful representation of the pain with a minimum of drawing. He uses the scale that is given in the instructions and does not elaborate or magnify his condition.

Interpretation of the drawing remains in question. Generally the drawing demonstrates a pain pattern that is local, referred, dermatomal, sclerotomal, or diffuse nonanatomical.

```
                              PAIN SCALE

        Instructions:                              _____ R.P.T.

        Use 0 to 10 scale

            0    No pain.
            1    Mild pain, which you are aware of, but not bothered by.
            2    Moderate pain that you can tolerate without medication.
            3    Moderate pain that is discomforting and requires medication.
            4-5  More severe and you begin to feel antisocial.
            6    Severe pain.
            7-9  Intensely severe pain.
            10   Most severe pain; you might contemplate suicide over it.
```

Activity	Comments	Location of pain	Time	0	1	2	3	4	5	6	7	8	9	10

Fig. 1-6. Pain scale.

PAIN SCALE

We use a pain scale (Fig. 1-6) for better communication between the patients and those treating them. Our scale is rated from 0 to 10. Zero is no pain at all, and 10 is pain that would be so bad that one would contemplate suicide. In general, any frequent pain over the grade level of 5 indicates magnification or expansion of the patient's painful syndrome. We have the patients grade their pain on a graph throughout the day. Pain that does not change during the day and does not go below a grade level of 3 with rest is suspected to be related to psychological problems, cancer, or disease processes originating in locations other than the degenerative spinal segment.

PHYSICAL EXAMINATION

A complete medical-physical examination of all regions of the body should be done before confining the examination to the spine. We do not deal here with the total physical examination, but confine our attention to the spine. As with any other musculoskeletal examination, we use the basic techniques of inspection, palpation, range of motion, neurological examination, and dynamic evaluation.

The back patient should disrobe completely to allow more complete inspection of the affected areas. The patient is observed as he disrobes to note the quality of movement. Patients will display their limitation of motion and pain responses, which should be consistent with the physical examination that follows. The patient is first examined standing, observing any abnormalities in posture, such as kyphosis or lordosis. Scoliosis or lateral curvature of the spine is particularly valuable to note. The skin must be closely inspected for any lesions such as hairy patches, cafe au lait spots, or birthmarks.

While the patient is still in a standing position, palpation of the spine, skin, and muscles is accomplished. We are looking for areas of tenderness, muscle spasm, and abnormalities in contour. Every joint of the spine and each extremity is actively and passively placed through a range of motion to note any limitation or pain. A general examination of the patient includes noting the strength of each muscle group, making a circulatory evaluation, taking a circumferential measurement of each extremity, and doing a thorough neurological evaluation. Details on a thorough physical examination can be found in other texts. A dynamic physical evaluation, as described by Robin McKenzie, is an important aspect of our evaluation. In this examination note is made of any changes in the patient's pain, muscle spasms, posture, and movement involving repeated motions of the spine, such as standing, sitting, and lying down. The premise for such an examination is that changes occur in the vertebral alignment and vertebral canal with each motion. A disc protrusion can be made more prominent or less prominent as the position of the spine changes. Trapped nerve roots can alter their position and produce changing symptoms with repeated movements.

The patient is therefore examined in each of the sitting, standing, walking and lying down positions, as he is asked to flex and extend his spine to the point that pain will allow. His spinal contours are studied and recorded. Any muscle spasm, list, malalignment, or tenderness is recorded.

The patient first ambulates and similar recordings are made. Particular note is made of any limp, spasm, or spinal posture that changes as the weight is borne on each leg. The patient then stands with his weight equally distributed on both feet and goes through an active range of motion in all directions as fully as the pain allows. The point at which the pain develops, and the maximal tolerable range of motion, are recorded in degrees in every direction. Once the patient experiences pain, he returns to the neutral position and then repeats these same motions to see whether it becomes easier with a repeated range of motion. Whether the pain extends more peripherally or "centralizes," is recorded, as has been pointed out by Robin McKenzie.

The patient then sits down, and his spinal range of motion is evaluated. Straight leg raising is done in the sitting position with the patient's attention distracted. This is later compared with straight leg raising lying in a supine position. The patient is not aware that a slumped forward sitting posture produces full flexion of the lumbar spine. This is part of the "foil the faker" tests.

The patient is placed in a supine position and does repeated knee-chest positions, each time returning to the neutral position. His pain is evaluated with each repetition, as was done when he was standing. The patient then lies in a prone position and accomplishes spinal extension maneuvers by doing a partial pushup–a "press-up" with the pelvis remaining on the examining table and the arms straightening as much as the pain allows. Again, spasm, list, and alterations in pain distribution are recorded. Palpation of every spinal segment is determined with light pressure and then with heavier palpation. In the sidelying position each spinal segment is placed through motion by progressively rotating the shoulders and pelvis in opposite directions while palpating the interspinous ligaments and spinous processes and determining the painful locations and responses.

Straight leg raising is also done in the supine position. Straight leg raising must be done in several ways for maximal value. This includes repeating straight leg raising with the knee bent, the ankle dorsiflexed, and with the patient's attention distracted. Internal and external rotations of the hip at the point of pain are also important. Details of straight leg raising tests and other evaluations of the spine can be found elsewhere. An examiner should be familiar with all of the spinal evaluation tests including the Hoover, flip, Faber, and Lasegue tests.

One of the most important reasons for the physical evaluation of low back pain is to obtain objective determinations of what produces and relieves the patient's pain and limitations caused by the disabilities. Some of these determinations are made from the range of motion, strength, and neurological evaluations. The remainder of the evaluation, however, is more time consuming and usually requires the aid of an orthopaedic assistant or physical therapist. The patient should be taken through activities of daily living, as well as many positions and exercises. We use a formal exercise obstacle course, which we have devised for this purpose (see Chapter 4). It includes evaluation of the patient while he is sitting, standing, walking, bending, lifting, pushing, pulling, climbing, and reaching. The therapist evaluates endurance while the patient is walking and while he is on a stationary bicycle. He can also be evaluated while jogging if he can jog. This is discussed in more detail later in the book.

We now have an extensive history containing all the details of the patient's past treatments and present pain. We have a physical examination and objective evidence of his endurance, pain-producing factors, and consistency in his physical capabilities. We have a dynamic evaluation giving us some idea how the spine changes with repeated activities, and we have some idea, too, of the emotional involvement with his disease.

DIAGNOSTIC TESTS

At the completion of the history and physical examination, the tentative diagnosis can be made. The next chapter deals extensively with the diagnoses we use in our back school. No further diagnostic testing may be necessary, if the patient has a fairly clear-cut presentation and can be placed into a specific category and treated successfully. The patient is placed in the back school and given the appropriate rest, mobilization, or exercise program and is observed. If he improves and returns to normal activities, no further diagnostic testing is performed. If, however, the presentation is less clear, or there are signs and symptoms of a potentially serious disease, further diagnostic tests are indicated. Also, if the patient does not improve with a trial period of back school, as would be anticipated, further tests can be done to confirm or correct the working diagnosis.

There are many diagnostic tests that can help us confirm our tentative diagnosis, which we obtained from our history and physical evaluation. The tests also help us rule out innumerable other diseases that are not primarily spinal problems. These are fairly standard in most spinal centers. They include routine x-ray films, a bone scan, an electromyogram (EMG), laboratory studies, a discogram, an epidural venogram, a myelogram, and a computed tomography (CT) scan. These diagnostic tests are well delineated in the literature and are not explained at this time. It is sufficient to say here that we are looking for destructive bone lesions, nerve root involvement, infections, tumors, arthritis, herniated lumbar discs, and spinal stenosis.

The simplest and safest tests should be done first. Simple x-ray films and laboratory studies are most helpful in eliminating possibilities such as cancer, diabetes, and kidney, liver, and other systemic diseases. X-ray films can demonstrate destructive lesions, spondylolisthesis, arthritis, and spinal curvatures. Since the vast majority of low back pain emanates from the degenerative segment, we need studies to evaluate the degree of degeneration of the lumbar segments. Flexion and extension views and lateral bending views of the lumbar spine can give us a great deal of information about the stability and normal functioning of the lumbar segments. If neurological damage is suspected, an EMG of the lower extremities and back should be done 2 weeks after the onset of pain.

In the past the most common procedure for diagnosing serious spinal conditions and evaluating herniated discs and spinal cord tumors was the lumbar myelogram. It does have some morbidity to its use and should not be used indiscriminately. However, if there is progressive neurological loss or severe incapacitating pain, and if surgery is being contemplated, then a lumbar myelogram can give a large amount of information. It carries with it the benefit of obtaining cerebral spinal fluid, which additionally helps to identify intraspinal lesions, such as tumors. The CT scan has recently been developed for spinal conditions. With the use of sagittal reconstructions and 3-mm overlapping cuts, one can obtain more information from the CT scan than from the lumbar myelogram. The CT scan does not require an invasive technique like the myelogram does with the use of a lumbar puncture. The CT scan does require approximately the same amount of radiation and has minimal or no morbidity. It not only evaluates the disc, but also the soft tissues. Spinal stenosis is readily identified. The condition of the facet joints and course of the spinal nerves can all be clearly identified with the CT scan. The epidural venogram and discogram are less valuable tests and thus are used less often. Both are invasive, requiring needles placed in the spinal canal and the disc. Contrast materials are used, and x-ray films are taken. The response of pain to the discogram can be helpful in localizing and verifying the source of the patient's pain.

There are times when all of the previously mentioned evaluations and tests do not reveal the source of a patient's pain. These are usually individuals who have had multiple spinal surgeries, who are chronic pain patients, or who have several different diseases going on at the same time. Such patients may require an inpatient evaluation by a multidisciplinary team.

We may need even more extensive information about this patient's pain and its aggravating and relieving factors. Does the patient's pain go away with bed rest? If he knows that it does, this is a strong indication that there is some mechanical factor involved. If it does not, bed rest should be prescribed, preferably in the hospital, under direct observation. He should be kept there until his pain subsides. He should be under the direct observation of a therapist, and be either in the hospital or be very extensively educated by the outpatient back school before being sent home and then followed up closely by telephone. The patient stays in the position that is most comfortable. If he has become pain free, we attempt to increase activity while maintaining freedom from pain with back school or a flexion body jacket. If he has not become pain free after 24 hours of bed rest, allowing only bathroom activities, we then place him on a thick foam mattress with a hole cut out for the use of a bedpan. The patient is log-rolled as though he had a fractured spine. If he is still not pain free within another 24 hours of this treatment, various anesthetic blocks can be instituted. We are again assuming that this patient has had x-ray films, laboratory studies, and possibly bone scans, venograms or myelograms, or EMGs that have not demonstrated significant pathology. At this point, if we feel from our evaluation that this is a facet syndrome, then a facet block for diagnostic purposes is performed. If we feel that it is more of a nerve root irritation syndrome, then an epidural block is performed.

In doing and evaluating these blocks, it is essential to realize that they cannot just be relegated to a third party to perform. They are best done by the major treating physician who is familiar with the patient's pain patterns, pain tolerance, and aggravating and relieving factors. The patient should have had the full physical evaluation mentioned previously so that the assessment can be repeated after the injection during the anesthetic period. We use a long-acting anesthetic and then place the patient through the obstacle course and determine whether or not we have changed the patient's abilities and decreased the pain for an appropriate amount of time for the anesthetic used. Short-acting anes-

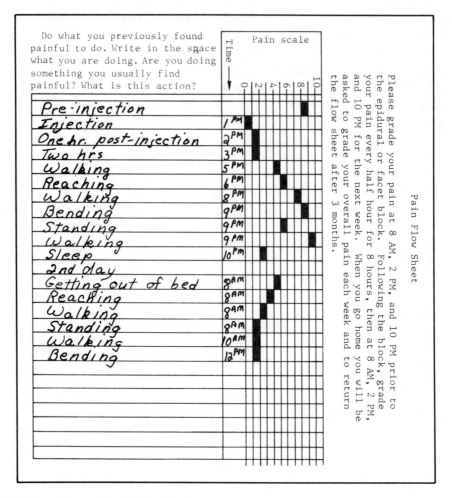

Fig. 1-7. Graph for recording pain after injections.
From White, A.H.: Evaluation of the chronic pain patient. In American Academy of Orthopaedic Surgeons: Symposium on the lumbar spine, St. Louis, 1981, The C.V. Mosby Co.

thetics and saline solution can also be used, if repeated blocks are required. A graph is used for the patient to record his pain for 24 hours prior to any injection, and then for 24 hours afterward (Fig. 1-7).

If these isolated one-time blocks and continued bed rest still have not relieved the patient's pain, we are faced with doing other diagnostic blocks.

THE INDWELLING EPIDURAL BLOCK

An epidural catheter can be placed through the sacral or lumbar route. Special needles and anesthetic trays are provided for these techniques. The needles have the opening arranged so that the catheter comes out at an angle to the tip rather than straight out the tip of the needle. Thus the physician can direct the catheter in any direction (Fig.

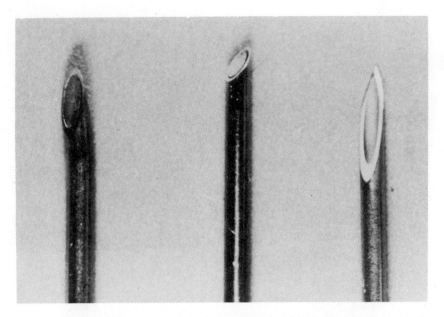

Fig. 1-8. Needle tips allow variable placement of catheters. Blunt tips make dural penetration less likely.
From White, A.H.: Evaluation of the chronic pain patient. In American Academy of Orthopaedic Surgeons: Symposium on the lumbar spine, St. Louis, 1981, The C.V. Mosby Co.

1-8). There is a slight chance of penetrating the dura through the lumbar route and thus placing the anesthetic within the dura and obtaining a spinal block. This brings out the necessity of doing these blocks in the hospital where there is good resuscitation equipment. There is much to be said for having an anesthesiologist place these catheters.

The monitoring after the anesthetic is instilled can also be done in a recovery room or emergency room situation where close monitoring is possible. The patient should not be left alone under a partial or complete spinal block. We have a therapist in close contact with the patient throughout the blocking procedure. Once we have verified the location of our catheter by x-ray films (Fig. 1-9) and we have achieved the initial block, we allow the patient to ambulate under direct supervision and return to his room.

The needle is placed in the lumbar route in the same form as a lumbar puncture. A hanging drop or air acceptance test is used as the needle is advanced to the epidural space. When the needle reaches the epidural space, air will be accepted freely and no cerebral spinal fluid is returned with aspiration. We then use a few drops of water-soluble contrast medium to verify the position in the epidural space. The catheter is advanced through the needle. The needle is then removed and the catheter securely taped to the skin (Fig. 1-10). Extreme motions of the trunk can dislodge or kink these catheters quite easily. The margin of safety for this displacement or kinking is much greater in the sacral route than in the lumbar route. This is because the catheter in the lumbar route is only an inch or two within the vertebral canal, whereas the catheter in the sacral route is many inches within the canal and could not be pulled out of the canal without extreme motion of the spine. At

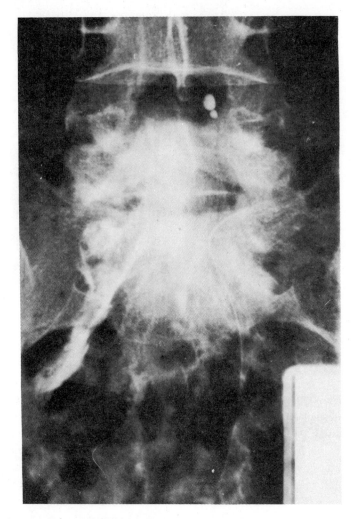

Fig. 1-9. Location of catheter verified by x-ray film.

From White, A.H.: Evaluation of the chronic pain patient. In American Academy of Orthopaedic Surgeons; Symposium on the lumbar spine, St. Louis, 1981, The C.V. Mosby Co.

any time throughout the procedure, a second injection of water-soluble contrast medium can verify the position in the canal. It is a good idea to do this at the end of the procedure as well as at the beginning.

Through the sacral route, the needle is placed just as it is with any sacral epidural block. A large-bore needle, however, is necessary instead of the 22-gauge needle we usually use for routine one-shot sacral epidural blocks. When the needle is felt to be adequately placed under local anesthetic, the catheter is threaded through the needle. If pain is experienced while passing the catheter, a small amount of ½% lidocaine (Xylocaine) is used within the epidural space. The catheter can be advanced well into the

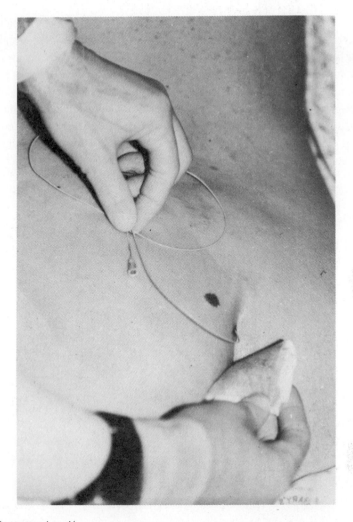

Fig. 1-10. Catheter taped to skin.
From White, A.H.: Evaluation of the chronic pain patient. In American Academy of Orthopaedic Surgeons: Symposium on the lumbar spine, St. Louis, 1981, The C.V. Mosby Co.

lumbar canal. A small amount of water-soluble contrast material will then display the level and location of the catheter and the anticipated distribution of the anesthetics, which will eventually be placed in the same volume. It is difficult to readjust the position of the catheter using this technique. The needle is removed and the catheter again taped securely to the skin and to a small empty syringe taped to the patient's flank. Do not pull the catheter back through the needle once it is in the spinal canal. It can be sheared off.

The sequence of injected solutions is a matter of personal preference. In general, the first anesthetic should be short-acting in case there is a complication. We use 1% chloro-procaine (Nesacaine) for the first injection. The patient and the physical therapist record the anesthetic response, the pain response, and the patient's physical capabilities. Depending on the results of the first injection, the second one could be normal saline solution or a longer-acting anesthetic such as bupivacaine (Marcaine). We are usually able to gather enough information during the day so that we rarely leave a catheter in place through the night. With the catheter in place, the patient is able to ambulate, climb stairs, and go through the obstacle course, which he previously went through for pain evaluation. We have had no complications with any of these blocks, but the potential complications are epidural hematoma, infection, spinal anesthetic with associated respiratory arrest, allergy to contrast medium or anesthetic, and dural penetration with cerebral spinal leakage.

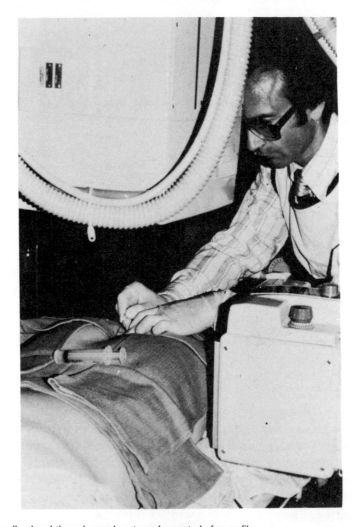

Fig. 1-11. Needle placed through sacral route under control of x-ray film.
From White, A.H.: Evaluation of the chronic pain patient. In American Academy of Orthopaedic Surgeons: Symposium on the lumbar spine, St. Louis, 1981, The C.V. Mosby Co.

SELECTIVE NERVE ROOT BLOCKS

When you want to more accurately localize the involved nerve root, selective nerve root blocks are helpful. The previous indwelling epidural blocks almost inevitably involve more than one nerve root and possibly both sides. A selective block can be done by placing a needle outside the intervertebral foramen. This is done by anesthetizing the skin approximately four of the patient's fingerbreadths lateral to the midline and placing a needle through the skin, passing it just distally to the transverse process and directly to the intervertebral foramen. An anterior-posterior and lateral x-ray film or fluoroscopy can verify the position of the needle (Fig. 1-11). The patient's pain response is also helpful in placing the needle, as well as confirming that the associated nerve creates a pain pattern similar to the patient's initial complaints. The needle can be placed through the outer covering of the nerve and contrast material injected. Reports have been made to demonstrate that such injections of contrast material can show evidence of external compression on the nerve. There are naturally inherent dangers in injecting contrast materials in such locations.

Once the needle is accurately placed, short- or long- acting anesthetics can be used. The anesthetic response of the patient and the distribution of anesthesia help verify again the nerve that is involved. The main response that is looked for is the loss of the patient's usual symptoms corresponding to the length of time of the anesthetic. Serial injections, injections with various anesthetics, and comparison with saline injections help to eliminate the placebo effect and to identify pain that is not of a physical origin.

When doing a selective nerve root block on the S1 nerve root, it is necessary to place the needle through the posterior intervertebral foramen of the S1 segment.

DIAGNOSTIC SPINAL ANESTHETICS

The diagnostic spinal blocks are usually done by an anesthesiologist and are the classical spinal anesthetics. The principle is to test painful positions and activities that the patient experiences. Usually you are comparing straight leg raising, areas of tenderness, and position of the spine. These positions and degrees of straight leg raising are accurately documented before the anesthetic is given. A painful stimulus is also graded before the anesthetic. We try to find a stimulus that is approximately equal to the amount of pain that is produced by the positive straight leg raising. The painful stimulus we usually use is squeezing the Achilles' tendon.

The patient is then routinely given a spinal anesthetic by an anesthesiologist. The anesthetic dose is initially very small and the patient's neurological response to the anesthetic is monitored closely. The painful positions and straight leg raising activities are reproduced during each degree of anesthesia. A comparison is made between the depth of anesthesia, the anesthetic response, and the point at which the patient's clinical symptoms and signs subside. If the patient's straight leg raising pain disappears at the same point that the painful squeeze of the Achilles' tendon disappears, it is likely that the pain is of a physical nature, which can be treated and pursued on a physical basis, and that is encouraging. If, however, the patient continues to have his pain when he is numb to the waist and no longer feels the painful squeeze of the Achilles' tendon, there is concern that the pain is of a more central nature and will not respond well to physical treatment. The same method can be used in the Pentothal examination. The patient is given a dose of thiopental (Pentothal), which eliminates all pain and motion. Then as the patient awakens, he is tested with straight leg raising and painful squeezing of the Achilles' tendon to see if the clinical signs and symptoms return at the same time as the painful external stimulus of squeezing the Achilles' tendon.

Discograms are thought by some to be of considerable value in reproducing a patient's pain. The radiographical picture of pain with a discogram, although of some value, is not as valuable as the pain response. In this procedure a needle is placed into the center of the disc. This can be done either from a direct posterior approach passing through the dura, or passing laterally adjacent to the transverse procedure. Biplane fluoroscopy and image intensification are valuable adjuncts for this procedure. A 22-gauge spinal needle can be used in the skin and directed by changing the bevel of the needle as it is advanced, or a double needle technique can be used. A larger bore needle is placed to the outside of the disc, and then a longer, thinner needle is placed through the outer needle and into the center of the disc. Once the needle is in place, any number of solutions can be injected to create pain and relieve pain. Usually a contrast medium is injected. The pressure of the injections, as well as the irritation of the contrast medium, produces some pain. If this pain is severe and closely corresponds to the patient's usual clinical pain, you can more strongly consider that disc a source of the pain. A low dose of short-acting anesthetic is then injected, and the patient's pain subsides. Much of the time the contrast material and the anesthetics leak out of the disc into the epidural space. It may be the effect on the epidural space that is really causing and relieving the patient's pain. Complications are, of course, the same as they are for epidural injections. Additional potential complications are disc space infections and possible weakening of an otherwise normal disc.

FACET BLOCKS

The original facet block usually includes two or three joints and possibly two or three on either side. The facet block is diagnostic as well as therapeutic. Each injection is graded for the patient's pain threshold to the skin anesthesia. Each patient grades his pain from 1 to 10 early in the evaluation and becomes accustomed to using the grading scale of 1 to 10 throughout all of these evaluations. The pain threshold is based on the skin anesthesia with a 30-gauge needle. The response then to the spinal needle passing through the fascia into the facet joint is determined. Each facet joint is probed and the pain recorded. Each joint is then anesthetized and entered with an 18-gauge needle. Steroids may be used, if we are convinced that the pain pattern is being accurately reproduced by the probing of the joint with the needle prior to anesthesia. Thus, we find whether the patient has a low pain tolerance or a hypersensitivity to all needle placements. We also find whether he has one, two, three, or six facet joints that are acutely tender, or whether one is severely tender and the others normally tender. This leads us to a segment from which painful pathology may exist. It makes the facet joint strongly probable as the culprit.

A facet arthrogram may also give us an indication of the degree of deterioration of that joint capsule. The degree of pain relief and the length of time that the relief lasts are closely followed. If marked relief is obtained temporarily, more permanent procedures can be planned with the patient. It takes extreme organization to be able to adequately get to know the patient on an outpatient basis. There is opportunity in the hospital for the staff to become more familiar with the patient and his condition. The hospital stay is not a situation that simply involves prescribed bed rest and a daily visit by the physician. Pain must be evaluated, monitored, and recorded under all circumstances. Changes need to be made in the patient's environment and activities until the patient becomes comfortable. Medical alterations in the patient's condition are induced by injection procedures, traction, flexion body jackets, and manipulations. The response to these alterations in the patient's pain and function help us to define the degree and location of the pain, as well as to provide possible long-range therapeutic measures.

Summary

At the end of the evaluation of the chronic pain patient, we have usually found that the pain can be attributable to a variety of sources in any one individual. I attempt to explain to the patient these various sources and the approximate percentage of pain that I feel is coming from each source. The patient is told if he has a low pain tolerance or hypersensitivity of various structures in his lumbar spine. The facet joints and the pain that is coming from their inflammation is explained to him. Degenerative disc disease, scar tissue, and nerve root irritation are similarly described. The patient's psychological status and estimated degree of emotional factors that add to his pain are defined. The most appropriate treatment for each one of these sources of pain is outlined for him. A psychosocial, physical, rehabilitative, and possibly surgical plan is formulated to help the patient most rapidly and economically return to the least painful and most functional capacity possible.

2 CLASSIFICATION OF LOW BACK PAIN

There are many different classifications of sources of back pain. These originate from individuals who approach back problems from a specialty area. The anatomist will most probably classify back pain anatomically. The manual therapist uses a functional classification based on motion. The industrial physician bases his classification on social and industrial needs, which will not interfere with his legal and industrial position or his ability to get the patient back to work. There are also classifications that were developed before we had our current understanding of sources of low back pain. Some classifications are made according to geographical, cultural, and language differences. Thus we have such diagnoses as lumbago, spinal insufficiency, dysfunction, and derangement. All of these terms have great value in the context in which they are used and for communication by the individuals who use them. None of these classifications gives the user an indication of the etiology of the disease, its progression, or its severity.

The following presentation is our method of combining the clinical material we see at the back school with the experimental research and clinical studies reported in the literature. This gives us a reasonably good working classification of low back pain, which carries also an inherent understanding of the disease process we are treating. Such a classification makes it easier to provide therapy in a rational and understandable way. It gives us a basis of communication with all the professionals treating the patient. This is in contradistinction to the previous method of diagnosing all conditions as either a back strain or herniated disc, and then arbitrarily selecting one of the 10 or 20 favorite therapeutic modalities and applying one at a time until one works or they all fail.

FOURTEEN DIAGNOSES

1. Anulus tear
2. Chronic degenerative lumbar disc disease
3. Herniated nucleus pulposus without neurological signs
4. Herniated nucleus pulposus with nerve root irritation
5. Herniated nucleus pulposus with neurological deficit
6. Spondylolysis
7. Spondylolisthesis
8. Facet arthropathy
9. Scoliosis (postural strain)
10. Ankylosing spondylitis
11. Spinal stenosis
12. Iatrogenic back pain
13. Back sprain
14. Functional or psychological low back pain

There are many other obvious diagnoses, such as fracture, metastatic cancer, osteoporosis, and discitis, that are fairly clear and distinct entities. They are diagnosed by rather specific tests and clinical findings. They have little to do with back school and are not discussed in this book.

Anulus tear

One of the first abnormalities you see in grossly evaluating lumbar spines in the laboratory is a breakdown of degeneration in the anulus. This usually appears as fissures or tears in the posterior lateral aspect of the anulus. Such tears can be created in a laboratory setting by flexion and rotation of the segment under load. These tears can be seen and heard when they occur in a laboratory. In a clinical setting we frequently see patients who state that they heard or felt a tearing noise or sensation in their backs as they bent forward to pick up something. Many anulus tears, of course, go unnoticed, as evidenced by the fact that we all must undergo anulus tears and eventual disc degeneration as normal aging progresses. When the anulus tear is of sufficient magnitude, however, and extends to the surface or outer layers of the anulus, a pathophysiological mechanism is set into play, which creates the clinical picture of an anulus tear. There are pain fibers in the deeper structures of the anulus, but no circulation in that area in an adult.

As the tear approaches the surface of the anulus, vascularization, inflammation, and autoimmune responses can occur, and nerve endings can be simulated.

The exact mechanism of pain production is not known. The clinical picture that arises is certainly consistent with an inflammatory process accompanied by edema, posterior migration of the nucleus into the anulus tears, and resultant mechanical low back pain, which is aggravated with sitting and relieved with extension of the lumbar spine. These patients are usually able to stand and walk without much pain, although they might have a list in the lumbar spine and muscle spasm, which are protective mechanisms. Sitting is usually the most painful position, and these patients have difficulty standing up after sitting for a long period of time. Some patients even produce a herniated lumbar disc through these anulus tears after long periods of sitting, or by bending and lifting with the presence of an acute anulus tear.

Most of these tears resolve spontaneously without any treatment, if the patient avoids sitting and lumbar flexion. They resolve more rapidly with an extension type of self-mobilization of the lumbar spine.

Unfortunately, in the past, these patients have been diagnosed as having lumbosacral strains and they return to the same environment that produced their previous anulus tears. They produce further tears that result in chronic degenerative lumbar disc disease or in a frank herniated lumbar disc. These categories are discussed in the next section.

Chronic degenerative lumbar disc disease

After multiple anulus tears have developed, there are physical changes in the property of the intervertebral disc and its associated segment. There is dehydration of the nucleus and changes in the chondrocytes, collagen, and mucopolysaccharides. There is

Table 2-1. Findings in patients with low back pain and recommended therapy

Diagnosis	Mechanism of injury	Aggravating symptoms	Position of relief
Anulus tear	Lumbar flexion; loading and rotation	Flexion and sitting	Mobilize in extension; immobilize in neutral
Chronic degenerative disc disease and spondylolisthesis	Chronic abuse	Heavy spine activity	Immobilize in neutral
HNP[†] without nerve involvement	Flexion and rotation	Flexion	Mobilize in extension; immobilize in neutral
HNP with nerve involvement	Flexion and rotation	Any lumbar motion	Neutral; immobilize
Spinal stenosis	Chronic	Lumbar extension and walking	Flexion; immobilize
Facet arthritis	Lumbar extension and rotation	Extension and rotation	Flexion; immobilize in neutral
Ankylosing spondylitis	Spontaneous	None; present at rest	None
Scoliosis	Spontaneous	Heavy spine use	Mobilize and correct posture
Iatrogenic	Medical treatment, especially surgery	Continual or all activity	None
Psychological	Inconsistent	Inconsistent	Inconsistent

*ROM, Range of motion.
†HNP, Herniated nucleus pulposus.
‡SLR, Straight leg raise.
§EMG, Electromyogram.
‖CT Scan, Computed tomography.

Pain location	Physical findings	Positive tests	Treatment
Back	Spasm; list, ROM* decreased	None	Mobilize in extension or back school
Back; buttock occasionally	Spasm; list, ROM* decreased	X-ray film, narrow disc spurs	Back school; brace; inject
Back and buttock	ROM	X-ray film; narrow complete	Back school; mobilize; brace; inject; surgery
Back and leg	Spasm; list, ROM decreased, SLR‡ increased	X-ray film; EMG§; myleogram; CT‖ scan	Back school; brace; inject; surgery
Back; buttock or leg	ROM, decreased SLR	X-film; EMG, myleogram CT scan	Back school; brace; inject; surgery
Back with radiation to leg	Extension decreased; rotation tender	X-ray film; facet block	Back school; brace inject
Back	ROM decreased; chest expansion decreased	Sedimentation rate; HLAW 27; x-ray films of sacroiliac joint	Medication; back school
Back	Posture abnormal	X-ray film	Back school; mobilize
Back and on leg	Variable	X-ray film; EMG; myleogram; CT scan	Rest; pain control
Inconsistent	None; objective	Psychological tests	Psychological treatment

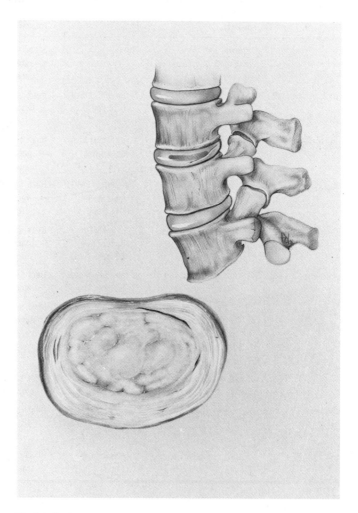

Fig. 2-1. Anulus tear.

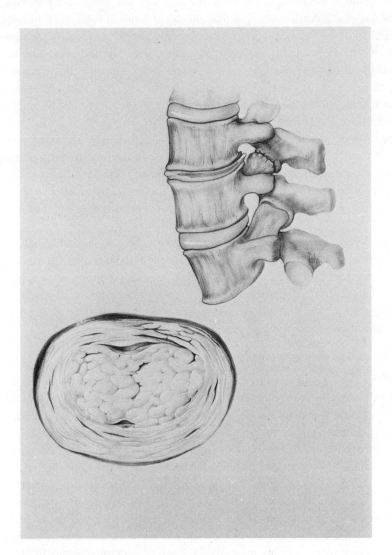

Fig. 2-2. Chronic degenerative lumbar disc disease.

alteration in the motion of the segment, less separation of the vertebra, less support of the segment, and instability. In rather gross terms, the disc eventually begins to look like a sack of mush, which fails to give support to all elements of the segment.

These changes can lead to alterations in the alignment of the facet joints and progressive alterations in the articular cartilage and capsule. The bone of the end-plates and vertebral margins undergoes changes that ultimately result in osteophyte formation. The anulus and all of the ligamentous structures become altered. Eventually the neurological contents of the vertebral canal may undergo compression. The clinical entities that can be produced by all of these changes are numerous. The diagnostic classification category could well be called the chronic degenerative lumbar segment. Many other names have been given to the clinical picture that this produces, such as lumbar insufficiency, spondylosis, instability, and arthritis.

The clinical picture that is produced by the previously discussed pathological changes is usually that of pain brought on with abuse of the lumbar spine. There may be occasional sudden catching pains in the low back. There is usually stiffness in the morning and then a period of relatively normal activity with minimal pain. After several hours of heavy use of the lumbar spine, or abusive positioning, pain develops that can last for hours.

Many forms of treatment help this type of pain, including antiinflammatory medication and physical therapy modalities, from ice to heat to mobilization. Braces and corsets allow increased activity with less pain. Injections are helpful during acute episodes. This type of pain goes on for many years until it eventually results in the patients greatly decreasing their activities of the lumbar spine, or until spinal stenosis develops. Spontaneous resolution of the pain can occur as the segment becomes fixed.

Herniated nucleus pulposus without neurological involvement

At any stage along the process of disc degeneration, as defined previously, the nucleus pulposus can escape through the anulus tears and enter the intervertebral foramen. A variety of clinical entities can be produced as the nucleus makes its journey.

Once the nuclear material comes in contact with the circulation, autoimmune responses can develop and be measured by laboratory tests. Inflammation and therefore pain can also develop. The nuclear material within the vertebral canal becomes a space-occupying lesion. This can cause direct mechanical effects on the neurological structures in the vertebral canal and the intervertebral foramen. Pain may result from direct physical pressure or chemical irritation. If the location of the nuclear material is such that the neurological structures are not involved, a clinical entity is seen that gives mostly back pain with no neurological or leg involvement. Such an occurrence is usually longer lived than the anulus tear and may create a permanent limitation in the patient's abilities and motions of the spine. A clinical picture simulating lumbar spinal stenosis can be produced, if the size and location of the nuclear material is appropriate. The initial inflammatory response may subside with time and leave a chronic space-occupying lesion in addition to the chronic degenerative lumbar segment disease. These lesions produce pain with specific positions and activities and produce relief with others. No neurological deficit exists.

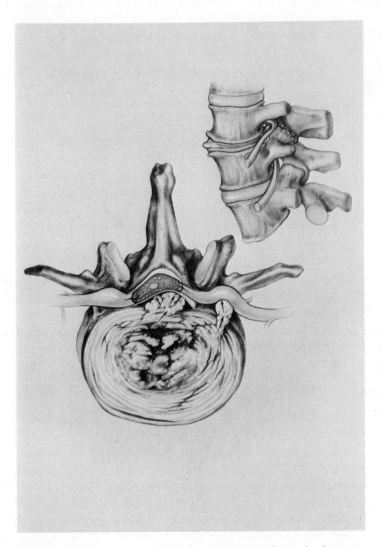

Fig. 2-3. Herniated nucleus pulposus with variable forms of nerve involvement.

Herniated nucleus pulposus with nerve root irritation

If the herniated nucleus pulposus material comes in contact with a nerve root, there is a certain degree of neurological irritation. This gives radiating leg pain at varying locations and degrees. Further motion or stretching of the irritated nerve accentuates this pain. There is frequently not enough irritation or compression of the nerve to produce neurological deficit. Therefore we see a clinical entity whose diagnosis and treatment are different from the preceding category and are frequently misunderstood because many physicians feel that herniated lumbar discs need to have neurological deficit. This entity can be severely painful and disabling. It can go on for years without showing neurological deficit. It can certainly alter the function and motion of the lumbar spine permanently.

Herniated nucleus pulposus with neurological deficit

The herniated nucleus pulposus with neurological deficit is the classical herniated lumbar disc that most clinicians recognize and on which most spinal surgeons operate. The herniated nucleus pulposus comes in contact with a nerve that becomes inflamed and painful initially. Neurological losses occur in the form of lost deep tendon reflexes, weakness, or sensory changes that are well known to all of us. The pain may totally subside and leave permanent neurological deficit. The neurological deficit may decrease or return to normal with time. There is usually permanent alteration of the mechanics of the lumbar spine, but surgery is only necessary occasionally. Nerves damaged by herniated nuclear material can be a source of long-range pain. Intraneural fibrosis can develop that acts as a focus or short-circuit, so to speak, for the existence of long-range neurological pain. Even after surgical removal of the offending nucleus material, the neurological damage can continue, being a focus of pain. Removing the offending herniated nucleus pulposus does not restore the vertebral segment to normal mechanical function. It is still a weak link.

Spondylolysis

Spondylolysis is probably a stress fracture that develops in the pars interarticularis of one or several of the vertebra. We see this entity mostly when we take x-ray films of an adult spine. No one is born with spondylolysis. When it develops, it usually creates pain. Any child or adolescent with back pain must be suspected of developing spondylolysis. It may not show up on x-ray films early, and therefore observation and further diagnostic tests, such as a bone scan, are frequently indicated. If not diagnosed and treated, it could be a source of chronic low back pain and lead to a need for spinal surgery. The spondylolysis alters the mechanics of the involved segment; as with any fracture, there is a painful local inflammatory process. It can heal, but once a nonunion of this fracture develops, we are left with a permanently altered segment. With time further alterations at the pars interarticularis can lead to neurological compression and nerve root irritation or neurological deficit. The altered mechanics of the lumbar segment can lead to the degenerative lumbar segment diseases listed previously. The instability of the segment leads to early degeneration and frequently to herniation of the adjacent disc.

Spondylolisthesis

As a direct extension of the previous category, spondylolisthesis can develop. All of the pathophysiology and symptoms created by the spondylolysis are then carried on in this category. As the segment becomes less stable, the vertebra slides forward, creating new types of pain emanating from the facet joint, supporting structures, and ultimately the nerve structures that are compressed and irritated. Although this entity can be found incidentally and may be painless, it frequently is the source of long-range low back pain and often leads to a need for surgery. As the segment passes through the stages of spondylolysis, degeneration, and neurological involvement, other categories of low back pain can be mimicked.

Facet arthritis

Many specialists in spinal disorders feel that most low back pain emanates from the facet joint. From the preceding description of the degenerating lumbar segment, you can see that there are considerable effects in the facet joint. Just as we see the disc go through a series of degenerating processes and end up "totally deteriorated," we see a similar series of events in the facet joints. The facet joints may even be the first area to undergo injury, with microfractures and capsular tears. The inflammation that occurs in the facet area is similar to traumatic inflammation of any other joint. This may occur with a single trauma, particularly that of extension and rotation. It may be a slow, more chronic inflammatory process related to segmental instability. The pain that develops can therefore be very transient or can develop into a long-range disabling condition. Pain is reproduced with certain motions and positions, especially lumbar extension and rotation. Neutral positions give relief. With advanced degenerative changes there may be malalignment, locking, catching, or partial subluxation of the facet joints. The facet capsule becomes stretched out and redundant, as does the synovial lining. This is frequently seen during surgery as a copious amount of whitish grey gelatinous membrane protruding both posteriorly out of the facet joint and anteriorly into the vertebral canal. During facet blocks and facet arthrography, the capsule accommodates several milliliters of contrast material, which can be aspirated and reinjected multiple times. There are frequently significant tears in the capsule and synovium, which allow the escape of contrast material into the vertebral canal. These findings can explain the source of a patient's pain with this condition. The malalignment and hypertrophy of the facet joints and their capsules not only create capsular distention, inflammation, and swelling, but can play a significant part in neurological compression in the underlying lateral recesses and intervertebral foramen.

Scoliosis and postural strain

The scoliotic curve has not been proven to be the source of low back pain. The alignment, mechanics, and stresses on the lower lumbar segments are altered by significant curves above that level. There may be more of a tendency to develop the degenerative lumbar segment when there are larger curves.

We see many elderly patients with no symptoms, who had scoliosis as children. As they get older and develop degenerated segments and arthritis, the curvature suddenly increases as much as 20 degrees in 1 year. They develop spinal stenosis in the lateral recesses and intervertebral foramina. When there has been a long fusion of the thoracic and lumbar spine, sparing only one or two lower lumbar segments, it only takes a few years of abusive activities with the back before significant degenerative pain develops. If there is a congenital spinal stenotic condition existing, the entire picture becomes much more incapacitating and painful. We also see a clinical entity that is frequently involved with scoliosis, which many professionals call postural strain. This can occur with scoliosis or any of a variety of postural extremes that cause a chronic, low-grade fatigue type of pain that changes rapidly with various forms of postural alignment, bracing, exercises, and manipulation. I am unable to give a pathophysiological explanation for this clinical entity. It may simply be a low-grade element of the chronic degenerating segment, or it may be simple strain or sprain, as we see on any other muscle-joint complex of our bodies when we are in an extreme position for a long period of time.

Ankylosing spondylitis

The pain of ankylosing spondylitis can mimic many of the other categories of low back pain. It is generally less mechanical (regarding position and activity) than most of the other disorders. Its location varies. Stiffness is frequent. The pathophysiology of ankylosing spondylitis is well known. The main thing that we must remember about ankylosing spondylitis is to remain aware of it so that if any of our treatments aimed at other diagnoses are not working for us, one of the first things we must do is test for ankylosing spondylitis. This should also serve as a reminder to look into all the other systemic and nonspinal sources of low back pain. Ankylosing spondylitis can go undiagnosed for many years, while the patient receives every other diagnosis and treatment known to medicine.

Ankylosing spondylitis is best confirmed by changes on x-ray films of the sacroiliac joints. These demonstrate sclerosis and obliteration of the joints produced by sacroiliitis. Late in the disease, the spinal segments show calcification along the longitudinal ligaments. Laboratory studies to help confirm ankylosing spondylitis involve the sedimentation rate during the acute phases of the disease and the HLAW 27 antigen, which is positive in most cases of active ankylosing spondylitis. The chest expansion of a patient with ankylosing spondylitis is eventually less than 1 inch.

Spinal stenosis

Spinal stenosis can occur as part of many other diagnoses of low back pain. It can be the end result of any of the categories already mentioned. There are many classifications within the category of spinal stenosis, ranging from fracture to Paget's disease. It is sufficient to say here that you are either born with a small capacity in the vertebral canal, or a small capacity develops with time and disease. When the capacity in the vertebral canal becomes too small, neurological compression occurs and can give a wide variety of symptoms. There can be selective nerve involvement with nerve root irritation or neurological losses. There can be collective nerve root compromise that can give only back symptoms with limitation of motion. Spinal stenosis underlies and is mistaken for many other entities, as it recurs in its various forms. If surgery is done for one of the other diagnoses of low back pain and spinal stenosis is not recognized as an underlying cause, the surgery frequently fails to correct the condition.

Spinal stenosis is easily diagnosed with a CT scan or a myelogram. Plain x-ray films do not usually confirm spinal stenosis, but ultrasound tests can strongly suggest it. When it becomes severe, there is obvious neurological loss with a positive EMG and a rampantly abnormal myelogram. Early in the disease, spinal stenosis can be very confusing and looks more like psychological or emotional problems because of the lack of objective positive physical findings. An anterior-posterior diameter of the lumbar vertebral canal at the L4 or L5 levels of less than 15 mm is presumptive evidence of spinal stenosis. At 10 mm there is absolute spinal stenosis and surgery is almost inevitable.

Iatrogenic

Iatrogenic may not be a fair term for this category. Medical treatments, especially surgery, are largely responsible for the patient's pain. The patients had some underlying degenerative segment disease or other diagnosis of low back pain before being medically treated. These medical treatments, however, carry with them certain risks and permanent changes. Every invasive diagnostic and treatment measure carries with it the risk of creating scar tissue, damaging neurological structures, or further weakening the structures of the spine. Arachnoiditis, intraneural fibrosis, extradural scarring, instability, and post-operative spinal stenosis are frequently seen. For the most part these are entities that cause permanent, chronic, painful conditions. Some of these are avoidable, but others are an inevitable risk of the diagnosis and treatment procedures.

Back sprain

Back sprain is probably the most common diagnosis used for back pain in the United States today. It is very difficult to discover what a back sprain is on a pathophysiological basis. It probably represents either an anulus tear or some form of chronic degenerative segment, which gives the patient temporary pain. The diagnosis is used because of a lack of more specific knowledge about the location of the pain. It is somewhat like lumbago, or low back pain of undetermined origin. I use this category mainly as a holding pattern when I am not certain of the underlying pathophysiology. With time the entity tends to sort itself out and fall into one of the more classical patterns. For example, the patient may come in with several recurring episodes of low back pain that do not fit any of the specific categories. The pain resolves each time, rapidly, and then an episode occurs that gives more buttock pain, then more leg pain, then positive straight leg raising, and then neurological deficit. We have been observing, of course, an atypical sequence of the degenerating segment, which resulted in a herniated nucleus pulposus with progressive neurological involvement.

It may be appropriate to use the term *back sprain* for entities that do not quite fit elsewhere. There may also be an entity of acute stretching trauma to the muscles and ligaments of the spine that can cause them to tear. This is similar to a sprained ankle. There can be hemorrhage, inflammation, and pain. This usually requires considerable trauma, although some clinicians feel that minor or lesser degrees of trauma can create muscular ligamentous pain. Many treatments have been aimed at these soft tissue forms of chronic back sprain. The diagnosis of soft tissue sprain, and its treatments, have not stood the test of time. They have not withstood the scientific process. No one has been able to reproduce any good clinical studies. There is no pathophysiological basis that has been proven or broadly accepted to explain significant chronic low pain emanating chiefly from muscular ligamentous structures.

I am spending more time on this subject because it is one of the biggest myths in the study of low back pain. It is one of the biggest misunderstandings that is passed on to generation after generation of medical practitioners. It is akin to the common cold being caused by drafts. If you have not gone past the belief in back sprain being a major cause of back pain by this time, you should stop reading this book and return to the scientific studies that have been the basis for everything discussed until this time. All the modern texts on the etiology, diagnosis, and treatment of low back pain fail to explain and frequently do not even mention back sprain as an entity. All the scientific studies that can be found in the literature fail to define or substantiate back sprain as a clinical entity. Back sprain seems to be an excellent place for practitioners to ''hide out'' when they have not been willing to really study the science of low back pain thoroughly.

Many times a practitioner cites one or two of his favorite studies, which were produced in some obscure journal or textbook. He latches on to that study as an answer to the source of low back pain. If we are truly going to be scientists and open-minded practitioners, we must adhere to the scientific process and subject such statements and isolated reports to a scientific double-blind process. There is never total agreement on anything, but there is general agreement in the literature on the spine that back sprain is a vague entity and that musculoligamentous abnormalities are not a major source of low back pain.

Functional or psychological low back pain

Our emotions play a large part in all disease processes. There are entire fields of medicine evolving that relate to the control of disease by emotional and psychological methods. All back pain patients have some degree of emotional involvement. Some back pain is entirely a psychological or emotional phenomenon. Thus all the categories of low back pain must take into consideration how much emotional or psychological involvement there is. It is very difficult to quantitate psychological involvement.

The low back area seems to be a common site for psychological problems to present themselves. There is a large amount of secondary gain from industrial and legal settlements involved in back problems. Many aspects of our culture tend to encourage psychological involvement. Studies have been done that demonstrate that the low back pain population has a higher degree of psychological problems than patients without low back pain. Other studies have shown that back pain is more severe and successes in treatment are poorer in patients with psychological involvement. Individuals with stress and emotional turmoil in their lives tend to have more low back pain and respond poorly to treatment.

We therefore use this classification of low back pain for patients who have a minimum of physical findings and a known large amount of psychological sources for low back pain.

SHORTCUTS TO CLASSIFICATION IN DIAGNOSIS OF LOW BACK PAIN

Although we advocate a complete history, physical examination, dynamic evaluation, accurate diagnosis, and appropriate studies and treatment, there is somtimes a need for shortcuts in identifying a patient's problem. It is necessary to capsulize the total concept of back care so that it is easier to understand and so that individuals who are forced into treating low back pain without adequate education or facilities can do so effectively. We therefore are including the following information as the shortcuts to diagnosis and management of low back pain. (See boxed material below.)

In reducing the low back pain patient's history to an absolute minimum, the most important information is the mechanism of injury, the aggravating and relieving factors, the location of the pain, and the response to previous treatments. Flexion injuries usually involve discs or end-plates. If the mechanism of injury is extension, the pain usually

---

ACUTE BACK PAIN ONLY

I. Dynamic (McKenzie) evaluation

A. Improves with extension
  1. Press-up and extension exercises
  2. Lumbar lordosis pillow for sitting
  3. General back school after pain free for 1 week
  4. Extension program with any recurrence
  5. Full flexibility program with maximum strength and range of motion (perhaps in a sports medicine facility) after completion of back school and 1 month free from pain
  6. Dynamic evaluation, if program ceases or fails
  7. Section on chronic low back or leg pain when plateau is reached and long-range low back pain continues

B. Improves with lumbar flexion
  1. Flexion exercises to use painlessly and progressively
  2. Extension avoided
  3. Basic back school
  4. Full flexibility and sports medicine program when pain free for 1 month
  5. Dynamic evaluation, if acute recurrence
  6. Chronic programs, if long-range low back or leg pain develops

C. Does not improve with either flexion or extension
  1. Immobilization, back school
  2. Facet block, if positive facet maneuver
  3. Epidural block, if positive disc or nerve root maneuver
  4. Body jacket, if immobilization relieves pain
  5. Bed rest, medication, and therapy
  6. Trial of mobilization
  7. Section on chronic low back pain, if above measures fail

CHRONIC LOW BACK PAIN

I. Previous section on acute low back pain

   A. Dynamic examination
   B. Facet block
   C. Epidural block
   D. Flexion body jacket
   E. Back school
   F. Mobilization

II. Extensive training and education

   A. Back school
   B. Industrial back school
   C. Sports medicine back school
   D. Ergonomics—environment and job change
   E. Long-range bracing and body jackets
   F. Repeated injections
   G. Diagnostic workup, if pain is still at an unacceptable level

III. Evaluation for chronic low back pain resistant to treatments I and II

   A. Flexion and extension x-ray films
   B. Bone scan
   C. EMG
   D. CT scan
   E. Venogram
   F. Myelogram
   G. Laboratory evaluation for arthritis and tumor
   H. Diagnostic blocks
   I. Psychological testing

IV. Surgery if treatments I, II, and III fail to relieve the pain, and evaluation demonstrates significant, correctable pathology in a psychologically stable patient

   A. Laminectomy
   B. Broad bilateral laminectomy
   C. Intertransverse distraction rod fusion
   D. Interbody fusion, posteriorly
   E. Interbody fusion, anteriorly

emanates from facet joints or foraminal stenosis. Similarly, pain aggravated by sitting and flexing is usually of disc origin, whereas pain from extension and rotation is usually of facet origin. Back pain is more frequently caused by facets, spondylolysis, anulus tears, and chronic degenerative segment disease. Buttock pain frequently is radiating pain from the facet or disc, but leg pain is usually neurological in origin, from spinal stenosis or herniated lumbar disc. Most mechanical sources of low back pain resolve with rest. Tumors, arthritis, and infections usually continue to be painful, even at rest. Extension treatment usually improves anulus tears and early disc degeneration. Flexion treatment frequently improves bulging discs, facet disease and spondylolysis. Proper mobilization and injections can improve most origins of spinal pain, except for tumor, infection, and fracture.

ACUTE BACK AND LEG PAIN

I. Rest, back school

   A. Bed—contour position
   B. Immobilization—back school
   C. Body jacket

II. Antiinflammatories

   A. Oral
   B. Epidural
   C. Intradiscal
   D. Intrathecal

III. Mobilization

   A. Trial of extension
   B. Trial of flexion

IV. Traction

   A. In bed
   B. Gravity hanging traction
   C. Intermittent physical therapy
   D. Body jacket

V. Section on chronic back and leg pain (next box), if treatments I, II, III, and IV fail to give relief within 1 month

CHRONIC BACK AND LEG PAIN

I. Treatment procedures listed in box on acute low back and leg pain

II. Diagnostic procedures

   A. EMG
   B. Diagnostic blocks
      1. Epidural blocks
      2. Selected nerve root blocks
      3. Facet blocks
      4. Intradiscal blocks
      5. Indwelling epidural blocks

   C. Myelogram
   D. CT scan
   E. Venogram
   F. Bone scan
   G. Laboratory

III. Surgery

   A. Laminotomy
   B. Laminectomy
   C. Broad decompressive laminectomy
   D. Consideration of fusion under special circumstances
   E. Distraction rod fusion

In a similar fashion, the physical examination can be generalized to come to a quick working diagnosis. Patients with neurological deficit or positive straight leg raising usually have herniated discs or spinal stenosis. Acute back pain with muscle spasm, list, or severe limitation of motion in most directions is caused by a major injury of the disc, such as a large anulus tear, a central herniated disc, fracture, or infection.

Low back pain of a relatively minor nature, which does not cause excruciating symptoms, major muscle spasm, or leg radiation, is usually related to the degenerative segment. This can be early disc degeneration, facet degeneration, or chronic degeneration and instability of an involved segment. The resultant back pain comes on after extremes of range of motion or periods of heavy use of the lumbar spine. There can be variable amounts of muscular and ligamentous contribution to this painful syndrome.

Therapeutic measures are applied to the diagnosis as derived from the mechanism of injury, historical factors, and physical examination. If the patient responds appropriately and rapidly, further diagnostic measures are not necessary and simple back school techniques keep the condition under long-range control. If success is not rapid, further diagnostic and treatment procedures are indicated. These can include diagnostic and therapeutic blocks and cortisone, an EMG, a bone scan, a myelogram, a CT scan, a body jacket, mobilization, psychological testing, and hospitalization. If a surgically correctable disease is found and conservative measures fail, surgery should be done as part of the rehabilitation process, rather than waiting for the patient to become progressively more debilitated before surgery. If surgery is not indicated and long-range disability is anticipated, the patient should be informed that changes need to be made in his occupation and his psychosocial environment to help him cope.

3 HISTORY OF BACK SCHOOL

In industrialized cultures we begin to experience back pain in our mid-30s. X-ray films and microscopic, chemical, and laboratory studies demonstrate that degenerative changes begin to occur in our spines at about that time.

Most low back pain comes from premature aging of the intervertebral lumbar disc and its associated lumbar segment. This process seems to be accelerated in industrialized countries by the exceedingly erect posture, by lack of useful range of motion of the lumbar spine, by incorrect bending, lifting, and sitting, and by many other as yet unidentified factors.

The overwhelming majority of low back pain patients can be treated successfully with very simple measures, such as rest, education, and training. With a little education as to the source of the pain, the patient can change his body mechanics slightly, do a few exercises, and make a small number of other changes in his activities and his environment, thus becoming the master of his back pain rather than allowing it to master him. The means by which this information is transferred to the patient has led to a whole new specialty of medicine and education that is commonly called back school.

In its strictest definition back school is an educational and training facility that teaches back health care and body mechanics to individuals to enable them to rapidly return to normal activity and to prevent further incidence of low back pain. In a broader sense back school encompasses early public education, specific education and treatments to all patients with all forms of low back pain, alterations of industrial sites and job descriptions, care of the patient in the hospital before and after operations, pain control, and the development of educational materials for the back pains of all segments of society.

For years physicians instituted preventive strengthening, flexibility exercises, and posture changes in patients with low back pain. This form of treatment decreased the episodes of patients' low back pain and gave them control over their conditions. If people were given back education and training in school as a part of health education, the incidence of back pain and the necessity for back surgery would be greatly reduced.

Booklets and pamphlets on bad backs have been issued to patients for many years, but the patients do not seem concerned or stimulated enough to study or use this information. When the patient's pain subsides, there is no stimulus to continue alterations in his bad habits, which have been so firmly fixed over the years. Changing your body mechanics is like learning a new dance. You cannot learn it from a booklet or a lecture. You must practice it, and it must become a natural habit pattern. This takes considerably more time than simply reading or being told how to do something in a different way. In this book we dissect adverse habit patterns and the means of correcting them.

Most patients who walk into the general practitioner's or general orthopaedist's office with back pain spontaneously recover within a few weeks. These patients obviously do not need any extensive back school training to get rid of their back pain. However, it has been shown that many of them would avoid recurrences and long-range back problems if they were given some prophylactic education at the first episodes.

DEVELOPMENT OF BACK SCHOOL CONCEPT

The beginning of back school can be traced to around 1958. At that time Dr. Harry Fahrni, who is now in Vancouver, Canada, was using the concept of back education for his patients. He realized that back pain was a controllable condition and developed many good techniques for resting the degenerating spine and then using body mechanics and back health education to control the back pain. He was one of the first to understand and elucidate the difference between the ground-dwelling and industrialized cultures. He demonstrated that ground-dwelling individuals did not develop degenerative disc disease and painful spines until the fifth or sixth decade compared to the industrialized cultures, which developed back pain in their mid-30s. He wrote articles and books demonstrating these principles. Dr. Fahrni trained physical therapists who have helped with the education and training of back pain patients.

Approximately 10 years later the Swedish low back school was developed. This back school is located in the Volvo factory in Sweden and mainly treats industrial patients. The Swedish approach to back school has mainly been one of group education to industrial patients who have been recently injured. This program has been very successful in returning patients to work.

In Toronto, Canada, Dr. Hamilton Hall has developed a group education back program. He and his colleagues give lectures to groups of back pain sufferers. Dr. Hall is evaluating the program and is finding that the great majority of patients are retaining the education and using it to control their long-range back problems.

My specific need for back school developed out of a general orthopaedic practice. We knew from the teaching of Dr. Fahrni and others that back pain was preventable and controllable. I knew from my personal experience with my own back pain and with back pain patients that we were able to shorten the length of each episode of low back pain and prevent future episodes of back pain with educational back health care training. In the beginning the physician dispersed the education. It took 2 or 3 hours of education on separate occasions. It was done at first with the use of pamphlets and anatomical drawings. We then made some audiovisual slides of stick figures and pictures of ourselves doing various daily activities as demonstrations, both properly and improperly. As we treated more and more back patients, the time required for teaching became overwhelming. We felt that patients did not learn as well in groups as they did on a one-to-one, eye-contact basis. Each individual had his own specific problems that required special attention. We therefore needed a means of giving stimulating education for specific problems in an economical way.

Physical therapists are already well founded in the basics of body mechanics and require little additional information to understand the basic principles of preventive back health care. The physical therapist therefore took over the job of the one-to-one training of each back pain patient. The therapist, too, became overwhelmed with the work and required better educational techniques. Thus we began to develop professionally produced audiovisual programs that could keep the attention of the patient and transfer the information in an understandable and entertaining format. These programs were developed to cover all the major specific problems of our patients. These include such things as anatomy and body mechanics for the office worker, the housewife, the pregnant woman, the athlete, and those engaging in sexual intercourse. Each of these audiovisual slides reinforced what the physical therapist had already attempted to teach the patient.

The question arose from the beginning whether we were getting the information across to the patient. We therefore had to develop some form of evaluation. We developed an obstacle course and a written test to determine how much the patient had learned and how well he was able to put it into effect. The statistics from our studies and others are listed in the following discussion.

BACK SCHOOL STATISTICS

Statistics regarding back school are very difficult to produce. It is much like demonstrating that good dental hygiene prevents tooth decay, or that smoking cigarettes is related to lung cancer. It takes many years and many population studies to produce proof. Nevertheless there is considerable information in the literature confirming that education is successful in decreasing expense, pain, and suffering from medical illness.

In August 1974, a white paper on health education was presented to the health care services of the Blue Cross Association. It was addressing the need of the health care system to contain rising health costs and ensure the quality of health care services. The feeling was that education can give the patient an understanding of his condition, and then better compliance by the patient can be expected in his treatment regimen. If the patient understands that it is his own health that is at stake, he will take some responsibility for his own health care. After all, who is going to be a better guardian of his own health than the one who really understands the condition and the consequences of physical abuse to the body? It concluded that patient health education should be encouraged and supported by their organization.

There have been many articles in the literature that substantiate that health education does, in fact, improve compliance by the patient and reduce costs. Katherine Healy in the *American Journal of Nursing,* in 1968, demonstrated that preoperative instructions to surgical patients resulted in early discharge from the hospital. Lawrence Egbert in the *New England Journal of Medicine,* in April 1964, showed how preoperative education could reduce postoperative pain and the need for narcotics postoperatively. Leona Miller in the *New England Journal of Medicine,* in June 1972, showed that education caused a decrease in emergency room use by diabetics. Peter Levine in the *Annals of Internal Medicine,* 1973, gave some interesting specifics with regard to cost reduction by education in the hemophiliac patient. With education the days of inpatient hospitalization declined from 432 to 42. Outpatient visits per patient decreased from 23 to 5.5 and a total cost per patient went down 45%. In the *Journal of the American Medical Association,* in 1978, R.L. Kaye demonstrated reduced costs and better health care in patients with rheumatoid arthritis because of the education given them.

All of the previous articles verify what we have similarly experienced with medical problems such as tuberculosis, polio, and scoliosis; that is that education and prophylaxis can prevent many diseases. Low back pain is preventable, and if it occurs, it is controllable by education and training. A patient can develop an understanding of his disease, take responsibility for it, and then to a large extent control his pain. Thus we have developed the concept of back school.

Back school has been proven successful in many areas of the world. Table 3-1 demonstrates a comparison of the three back schools for which we have statistics at this time. Although the populations of each of the back schools are different, the success rates are all high. There is great satisfaction with the program — between 75% and 96%. The people who do not seek further attention range from 70% to 89% and the patients who find that their pain is at an acceptable level after taking back school are from 80% to 90%.

Industries are just beginning to institute back school programs and produce statistics. In one industrial program 39,000 employees of the Southern Pacific Transportation Company were taught back health care and protective body mechanics. The following year there was a 22% decrease in back injuries and a 43% decrease in lost time in one single aspect of that industry. There was over a $1 million savings that year.

Therefore we have personal and statistical evidence that back education and training is working for the patient, the physician, and industry. Industry continues to expand its education to employees before beginning employment. Many industries are already giving daily back health reminders and reinforcement. Safeway has instituted an international back protection project that involves the employees as well as their families in back education and exercise. They have developed what they call the "squat team," which is individual and group competition for the length of time individuals can hold a wall slide. They give prizes, such as vacations, to the winners. The record for a wall slide in their industry is now over 3 hours. They provide literature in the employees' pay envelopes, and they give out bumper stickers, posters, and T-shirts. They teach the straight back bend as a means of reducing their most common injury, which is in the warehouse and

Table 3-1. Statistics of three back schools' success*

	California Back School	Volvo factory	Toronto Back School
Patients satisfied with program	94%	75%	96%
Percent of patients not seeking further treatment	89%	86%	70%
Acceptable pain level in patients	95%	80%	80%

*From White, A.H.: Low back patient goes to school. In American Academy of Orthopaedic Surgeons: Symposium on the lumbar spine, St. Louis, 1981, The C.V. Mosby Co.

involves loading and unloading from under low racks. This type of program is now being expanded to the Red Cross.

Many industries are requiring back school and obstacle courses to be given to employees before beginning any work. Special training is given for jobs that require continuous heavy bending and lifting. Remedial back school is required of employees who have a new back injury before they can return to their usual work. If back injuries are not resolved within the usual anticipated week or two, the employees are sent to a spine center where a multidisciplinary diagnostic and treatment program is instituted before the employees develop long-range disability habits. This is a complicated psychological, social, and physical rehabilitation science, about which many books and articles have been written. We delve into this somewhat further in Chapter 5. Most of the industries with back programs have audiovisual presentations that workers in high-risk jobs must attend on a yearly basis. Safety trainers are taught to produce and deliver these prophy-lactic back health care programs. They develop their own style of presentation, which frequently includes tests for the employee as an indication of how much of the information is being retained and used. It seems to be important who delivers the education and training to employees. We see greater success when the training is given by fellow employees who are well accepted and respected by the trainees.

4 BASIC BACK SCHOOL

Back school was originally devised to educate the back pain patient in proper body mechanics and back health care. As the back school advanced into other areas, it became a diagnostic tool with the use of the obstacle course. It became a management tool for the physician to help his patients before and after trials of body jackets and braces, injection procedures, manipulation therapy, and surgery. Thus the standard outpatient back school has become a total outpatient management, diagnostic, and treatment center. It can be an irreplaceable tool for the physician in managing low back pain patients.

Basic back school, as we use it, calls for three visits in 3 weeks, with a recheck in 1 month. Each visit requires 1½ hours of practice and demonstration time. The nature of the back pain and sciatica can alter the length of any training session. We use the three visits to teach the coordination needed to apply protective body mechanics to daily activities.

Information is presented to patients in a variety of ways. These include didactic instructions, audiovisual presentations, and practice sessions. Some of these sessions are given in groups, but ability to comprehend and use proper body mechanics is tested individually. In general we prefer using a one-to-one educational technique because each individual's specific problems are unique. We feel that teaching body mechanics is like teaching dancing. You cannot learn to dance from a book or diagram. You must get in and participate on a one-to-one basis. When audiovisual materials are used, they simply reinforce what the patient has been taught by the instructor. There are no more than 15 minutes of audiovisual time in each hour of back school.

DAY ONE
History
Physical evaluation
Obstacle course
Treatment planning
Education in anatomy
Protective body mechanics and posture
Practice rest positions and exercises

DAY TWO
Evaluate progress
Teach body mechanics for daily living and
    job-related activities

DAY THREE
Evaluate progress
Retake obstable course
Train in body mechanics for sports and heavy
    labor or other specialized activities

DAY FOUR
Recheck day
    Physical evaluation
    Answer questions

DAY ONE

Day one of back school (see boxed material on p. 50) includes an interview with the patient, discussing his home, job, and specific needs or biomechanical problems involved in his diagnosis. It also includes a physical examination. If there is no neurological involvement or contraindication, the obstacle course follows. The back school physical evaluation (Fig. 4-1) is performed to assess the acuteness of the condition, consistency of the symptoms, and whether obstacle course or exercise training may be safely performed at this time. An evaluation is made on the first and last days of back school and on the 1-month follow-up visit. For those patients with acute symptoms, the evaluation is performed on an every-session basis to assess change, progress, and whether the next step of back school can be initiated.

Positive findings on any two of the following preclude the patient from the obstacle course and exercise period, as well as heavy lifting:

1. Straight leg raising tests
2. Crossed straight leg raising
3. Spasms causing marked limitation of lumbar flexion range of motion
4. Leg sensory loss
5. Leg weakness

If only one of the five findings is present, the patient is allowed to do the obstacle course an exercises under close observation, but is not allowed to do any heavy lifting.

The obstacle course measures the patient's performance on a standardized form and is used to create individualized instruction and training programs. Activities such as sitting relaxed, sitting to fill out forms, standing, walking, reaching, bending, kneeling, lifting, twisting, sidelying, pushing and pulling, going over and under obstacles, and resting postures in bed are tested. Any deficiency in these activities is scored and measured against accepted protective body mechanics concepts. An exercise tolerance test may be given on an exercise bicycle or by a timed wall slide, partial sit-up, or distance ambulated. The following pages outline the specific mechanism by which the obstacle course is given and graded.

The obstacle course

The goals of the obstacle course are

1. To identify repetitively performed postures or motions that produce pain or raise questions concerning the stated diagnosis
2. To provide a measurement device with a standarized scoring system that compares the performance with a like population of the same diagnosis, and each days' performance is scored to measure progress
3. To provide a training area for demonstration and practical application of the body mechanics theory presented
4. To provide a problem-solving area where patients may demonstrate and correct specific job-related body mechanics problems

We must assume that the performance closely follows the patient's normal habit patterns.

GOALS

Therapist

Obtain present and past history (Chapter 1)
Establish physical evaluation
Obtain functional screening (Chapter 1)
Obtain obstacle course rating
Establish program sequence and plan

Patient

Understand mechanisms causing pain
Understand resting positions for lying, sidelying, sitting, riding in a car, and for short periods of
    standing work
Understand first aid measures in case pain worsens
Demonstrate and discuss correct performance of exercises

SCHEDULE

Time (minutes)	Goals	Methods	Materials presented	Evaluation
15	Fill out history and billing forms	Patient	History form, pain drawing, billing form	Secretary for completeness
10	Past history, historical highlights and significant complaints identification	Therapist interview	History form, pain drawing, past history questions	Therapist review
10	Determine significant precautions and level of recovery	Physical evaluation, posture photograph	Physical evaluation form, posture photograph	Therapist examines patient
20	Obstacle course rating	Patient performs obstacle course	14 motions on obstacle course	Therapist grades obstacle course performance
10	Program planning	Discuss with senior physical therapist	History, physical evaluation results, obstacle course results, photograph, cooperation level	Senior physical therapist determines level and progression
10	Understand mechanisms that cause pain	AV-anatomy lecture, demonstration and patient feedback	Anatomy, concept of spine position and pain	Patient discusses spine position and pain
15	Understand positioning for pain relief	AV-lecture demonstration and patient feedback	Posture, positions of standing, sitting, and lying down, first aid	Patient practical demonstration and patient discussion

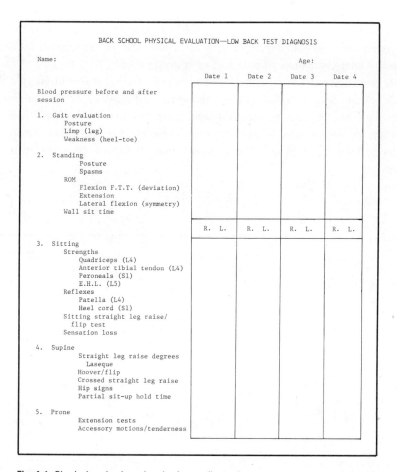

BACK SCHOOL PHYSICAL EVALUATION—LOW BACK TEST DIAGNOSIS

Name: Age:

	Date 1	Date 2	Date 3	Date 4
Blood pressure before and after session				

1. Gait evaluation
    Posture
    Limp (leg)
    Weakness (heel-toe)				

2. Standing
        Posture
        Spasms
    ROM
        Flexion F.T.T. (deviation)
        Extension
        Lateral flexion (symmetry)
    Wall sit time				

	R. L.	R. L.	R. L.	R. L.

3. Sitting
    Strengths
        Quadriceps (L4)
        Anterior tibial tendon (L4)
        Peroneals (S1)
        E.H.L. (L5)
    Reflexes
        Patella (L4)
        Heel cord (S1)
    Sitting straight leg raise/
        flip test
    Sensation loss				

4. Supine
        Straight leg raise degrees
        Laseque
    Hoover/flip
    Crossed straight leg raise
    Hip signs
    Partial sit-up hold time				

5. Prone
        Extension tests
        Accessory motions/tenderness				

Fig. 4-1. Physical evaluation—low back test diagnosis.

During patient performance it is important to observe the resting postures assumed between motions. Resting positions with exaggerated lumbar lordosis are not correct. The following resting positions are acceptable and are to be encouraged: pelvic tilt; placing one foot on a box, stool, or chair; wall leaning; and sitting in a reclining position.

Exaggerated lumbar lordosis during lifting, carrying, reaching (out or overhead), returning upright from a bend or squat, or twisting is observed, scored, and discouraged. Note at which point during a motion the exaggeration occurs so that a protective substitution motion or pelvic tilt may be initiated.

Complaints of pain are to be noted and observed for the exact point of motion that initiates the pain. Note whether the spine is flexed or extended, lordotic, and loaded with weight. Also note whether the same motion performed during another task produces the same pain. The significance of pain is unclear unless it is consistently produced with the same motion, many tasks. Complaints of pain are most significant if occurring during hyperlordotic posture, initial forward flexion, terminal forward flexion, lifting or carrying a weight associated with the first three, initial hyperextension associated with returning from bending, and terminal hyperextension associated with reaching out or overhead to a high shelf. Other complaints of pain are, of course, noted.

The obstacle course is designed to be physically taxing. It should provide an early indicator of endurance, especially for the abdominal and quadricepts mechanisms. It also provides the basis for teaching practical application of protective body mechanics. This training may be compounded by joint problems in the hip, knee, or ankle. An appropriate plan can be formulated to take into consideration all aspects of a patient's physical problems.

Name _____

GENERAL OBSTACLE COURSE

Observation date

	Score	Points	Score
Standing			
Posture	1	1	
No lordosis	2	2	
Knees flexed	1	1	
Sitting			
Posture	1	1	
Spine supported	1	1	
Buttocks tucked under	2	2	
Crouching			
Posture	1	1	
Flexibility	1	1	
Shoulders back and straight	1	1	
Forward bend			
Shoulder and foot position	1	1	
Straight spine	2	2	
Knee flexion greater than spine flexion	1	1	
Reaching			
Posture	1	1	
Straight spine	1	1	
Pelvic tilt, no lordosis	2	2	
Side lean			
Posture, no twisting	1	1	
Strong pelvic tilt	1	1	
Knee flexion greater than spine flexion	1	1	
Twisting			
Posture, free knee motion	1	1	
Shoulders and hips in line through twist	2	2	
No lordosis	1	1	
Push-pull			
Posture	1	1	
Pelvic tilt, no segmental motion	1	1	
Knees flexed and mobile	1	1	

Fig. 4-2. General obstacle course.

General obstacle course testing

The obstacle course normally follows the physical evaluation. The obstacle course is only done on patients whose physical conditions allow it. Generally this means negative neurological involvement, no straight leg raising or crossed straight leg raising signs, no leg strength loss, and no gross limitation of flexion caused by muscle spasms.

The obstacle course is scored on a form (Fig. 4-2) by circling the correct number score and crossing out the failed number score for each observation. These are the correct parameters:

	Score	Points	Score
Over and under			
Posture		1 1	
Shoulders back and straight		1 1	
Pelvic tilt	_____	1 1	_____
Lifting sequence			
Shoulder and foot position		1 1	
Pelvic tilt		1 1	
Straight spine bend		2 2	
Good knee flexion	_____	1 1	_____
Lying postures			
Supine			
Head and neck position		1 1	
No lordosis		1 1	
Slight knee flexion	_____	1 1	_____
Sidelying			
Head and neck position		1 1	
No lordosis	_____	1 1	_____
Prone			
Head and neck position		1 1	
Half sidelying, pillow under abdomen	_____	1 1	_____
Walking			
Head and shoulder position		1 1	
Pelvic tilt, no lordosis		2 2	
Knee position		1 1	
Foot position		1 1	
No limp	_____	1 1	_____
TOTAL		50 50	
	_____ %		_____ %

Further observations

Distance able to walk:_____ Time:_____

Stand comfortably _____

Sit comfortably _____

Comments:

The obstacle course begins with observation of the patient filling out forms.

Sitting—reclining position, no slouch, good beltline, low back support, knees flexed and above level of chair (Fig. 4-3).

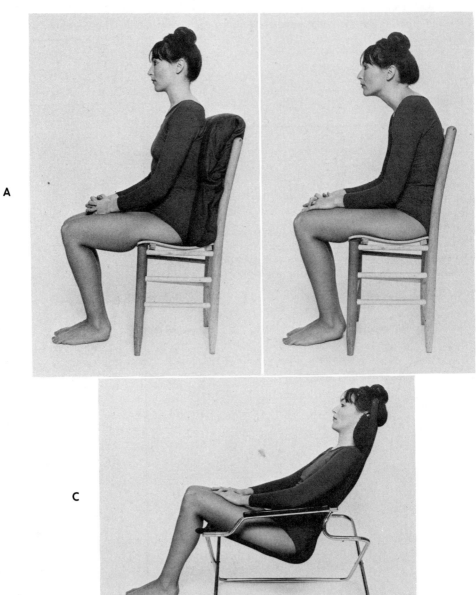

Fig. 4-3. Sitting. **A** and **C**, Right: low back supported and straight. **B**, Wrong: back bent.
From Mulry, R.C., White, A.H., and Klein, E.A.: The portable back school: a home study program for proper back care, St. Louis, 1981, The C.V. Mosby Co.

Standing in a resting fashion (Fig. 4-4) is observed during the physical evaluation and between obstacle course tasks. Observe carefully the habitual standing and relaxation postures.

> *Standing*—erect posture of shoulders, no lordosis, pelvic tilt, knees slightly flexed (Fig. 4-5).

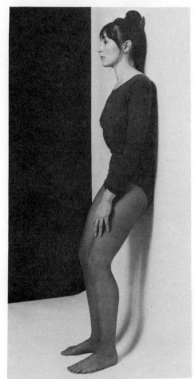

Fig. 4-4. Standing rest position. This is accomplished by leaning against the wall in the pelvic tilt.
From Mulry, R.C., White, A.H., and Klein, E.A.: The portable back school: a home study program for proper back care, St. Louis, 1981, The C.V. Mosby Co.

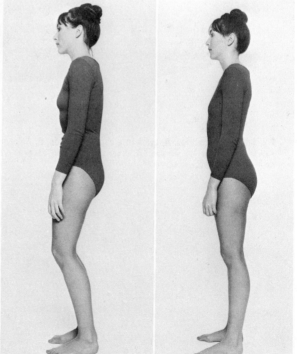

A

B

Fig. 4-5. Standing. **A,** Right: back straight, stomach in, buttocks under, and knees bent. **B,** Wrong: back swayed and knees straight (locked).
From Mulry, R.C., White, A.H., and Klein, E.A.: The portable back school: a home study program for proper back care, St. Louis, 1981, The C.V. Mosby Co.

Lying postures are evaluated during the physical evaluation. Ask the patient to demonstrate each.

Lying supine—head on low pillow, knees bent or elevated over pillows, feet on mattress (Fig. 4-6, *A*).

Sidelying—head on low pillow, knees drawn up and together, patient able to touch kneecaps with palms (Fig. 4-6, *B*).

Lying prone—no head pillow, pillow under abdomen or body, one knee drawn up.

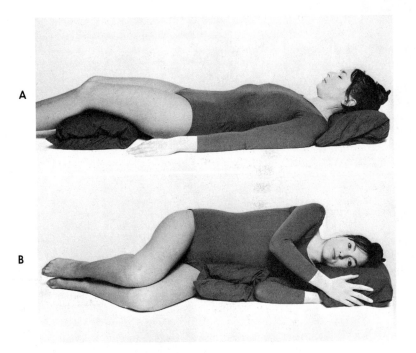

Fig. 4-6. Lying postures. **A,** Lying in a supine position. **B,** Sidelying (fetal).
From Mulry, R.C., White, A.H., and Klein, E.A.: The portable back school: a home study program for proper back care, St. Louis, 1981, The C.V. Mosby Co.

Next have the patient walk while you observe his gait posture.

Walking—ear over shoulder, no excessive lordosis, pelvic tilt, knees slightly flexed (Fig. 4-5).

Now walk to the obstacle course and begin testing by having the patient reach to a 78-inch high shelf for items.

Reaching—no lordosis, pelvic tilt, body C-shaped during reach (Fig. 4-7).

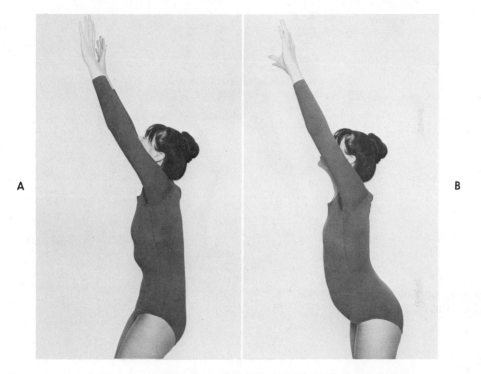

A   B

Fig. 4-7. Reaching. **A,** Right: back straight, stomach in, and buttocks under. **B,** Wrong: back swayed.
From Mulry, R.C., White, A.H., and Klein, E.A.: The portable back school: a home study program for proper back care, St. Louis, 1981, The C.V. Mosby Co.

Have the patient next demonstrate bending while holding the items grasped from the 78-inch high reaching test, and then placing the items on the floor.

Bending—knees bent to a greater degree than the spine, spine straight, no rounding of the shoulders, feet wide apart (Fig. 4-8).

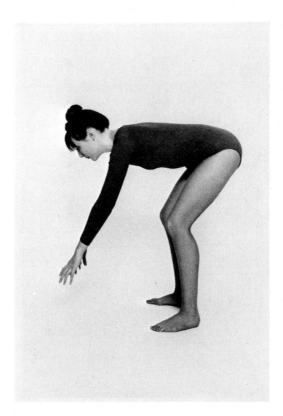

Fig. 4-8. Straight backbend: stomach tightened, back straight, and knees bent.
From Mulry, R.C., White, A.H., and Klein, E.A.: The portable back school: a home study program for proper back care, St. Louis, 1981, The C.V. Mosby Co.

Have the patient now move all the items on the 24-inch high bottom shelf to the 72-inch high top shelf. Reassess both bending and reaching as a combination motion.

Then have the patient crouch (Fig. 4-9), squat, or kneel down and place the items on the floor on the 24-inch high bottom shelf.

Crouching—one knee down (optional), back straight, stomach pulled in. Note flexibility of the heel cords.

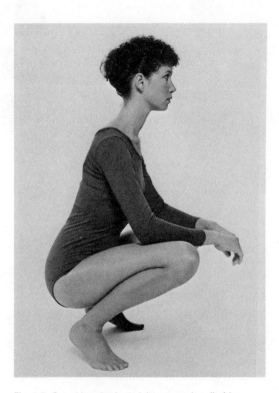

Fig. 4-9. Crouching: back straight, stomach pulled in.

Now have the patient unload the middle, 36-inch high shelf to either the shopping cart or a table. Note the twisting actions.

> *Twisting*—no lordosis, pelvic tilt, shoulders and hips in the same plane during twist, knees and feet free to move during twist (Fig. 4-10).

Have the patient return all the items to the shelf while you reassess the twisting.

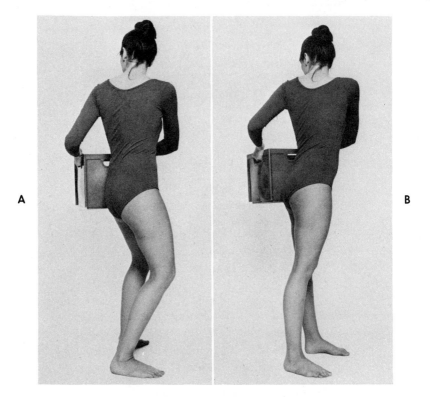

A   B

Fig. 4-10. Twisting. **A,** Right: turn shoulders, hips, and foot together. **B,** Wrong: feet planted and shoulders not in line with hips and feet.
From Mulry, R.C., White, A.H., and Klein, E.A.: The portable back school: a home study program for proper back care, St. Louis, 1981, The C.V. Mosby Co.

Have the patient lift a suitcase, tool box, or flight bag from a cluttered corner, under the table, behind a chair.

Side lean—no twisting, knees bent to a greater degree than spine, no lordosis, pelvic tilt (Fig. 4-11).

A   B

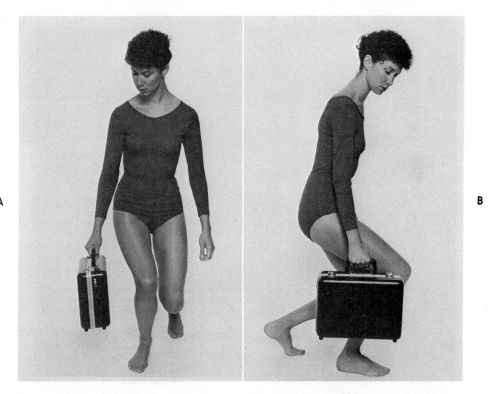

Fig. 4-11. Side lean: back straight, knees bent to a greater degree than the back.

Have the patient carry the item around the room and return it.

Assess lifting, remembering any precautions against heavy weights if indicated. Have the patient place two or three appropriately weighted grocery bags into the grocery cart.

> *Lifting*—feet wide apart, no lordosis, pelvic tilt on initiation and return from bend, straight spine, no rounded shoulders during bend, knee bend greater than spine bend (Fig. 4-12).

Lifting may also be assessed during the reaching-bending evaluation. Note that the load should always be close to the body.

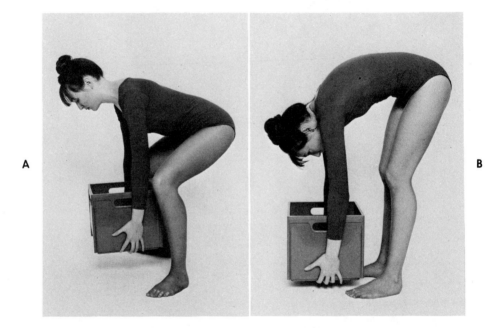

A   B

Fig. 4-12. Lifting. **A,** Right: back straight, stomach in, buttocks under, and knees bent. **B,** Wrong: back bent and knees straight.
From Mulry, R.C., White, A.H., and Klein, E.A.: The portable back school: a home study program for proper back care, St. Louis, 1981, The C.V. Mosby Co.

When the grocery cart is filled with either grocery bags or shelf items, pushing and pulling may be assessed. The patient pushes the cart out of the room and down a hallway, and then pulls the cart back over the same course.

> *Pushing-pulling*—no slouch, cart close to body, no lordosis, pelvic tilt, knees flexed and mobile (Fig. 4-13).

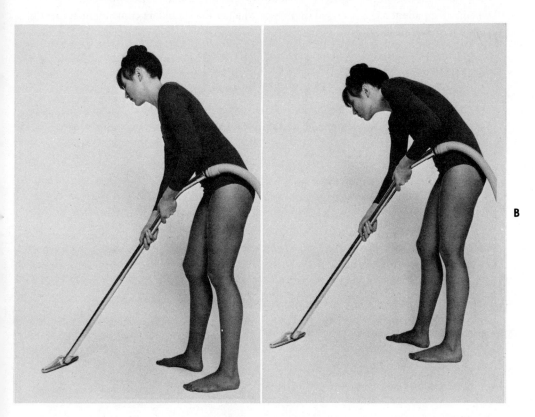

Fig. 4-13. Pushing and pulling. **A,** Right: back straight, stomach in, buttocks under, and knees bent. **B,** Wrong: back bent and knees locked.

From Mulry, R.C., White, A.H., and Klein, E.A.: The portable back school: a home study program for proper back care, St. Louis, 1981, The C.V. Mosby Co.

Finally assess bending and stepping over. Draw two cables across the room—one at a 24-inch height and the other at a 36-inch height, separating them by 48 inches. The patient steps over the 24-inch-high rope and then bends under the 36-inch-high rope. He repeats this process a few times. Note whether in stepping over, the legs are kicked out in front of the patient or to the side or back. In bending, note the posture on returning to upright. Is there a reversed lumbar-pelvic rhythm; that is, does the patient squat first and then raise the shoulders upright without performing spinal hyperextension? Observe whether the patient has a reversed rhythm or whether the shoulders come up first, creating spinal hyperextension.

Over—legs kicked out to front, pelvic tilt, no lordosis.

Under—knee bend greater than spinal bend, spine straight, pelvic tilt-squat on return upright, no hyperextension on return upright (Fig. 4-14).

This concludes the obstacle course. The scores should be added up and a percentage found and compared to the general population for that diagnosis.

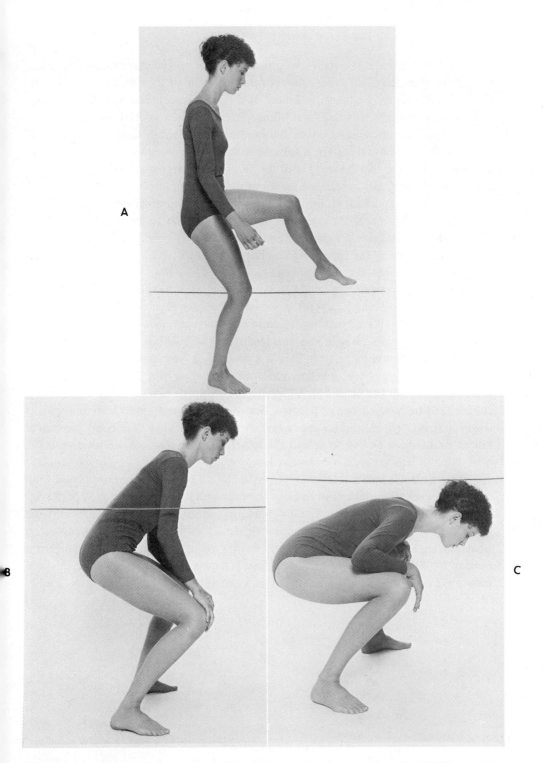

Fig. 4-14. Over and under. **A,** Over: back straight, stomach in, leg kicked out to front. **B** and **C,** Under: back straight, knees bent.

Patient instruction

The patient is told that certain rules governing spinal pain hold true for all diagnoses. Regardless of the diagnosis, your chances for spinal pain are increased by loaded positions, stooped forward positions, and those of sitting, especially in a slouched position. Hyperlordotic postures, twisting, and lifting, especially from stooped positions or at a distance from the body, are also potentially painful. All patients are taught the concepts of degenerative segment aging. They are taught that a disc loses its water content and decreases in size and that the stability of the intervertebral segment decreases. Facet and joint changes occur, and further breakdown of the segment follows. The low intradiscal pressure theory is explained. Protection of the spine and its segments through proper body mechanics is emphasized. Protection of the spine using the pelvic tilt (Fig. 4-15) is accomplished by abdominal tightening and bending the hips and knees to position the body instead of using the lumbar spine. The principles of body mechanics and their application to back health care are given.

On day one patients are taught that pain relief is accomplished by maintaining favorable resting positions, especially those where the spine is unloaded throughout all of their daily activities. If the dynamic McKenzie evaluation has demonstrated that mobilization or specific posturing is indicated, it is instituted. Otherwise all patients are instructed in the contour position for resting. This is a position of lying supine with the hips and knees flexed, using a pillow or bolster under the knees. Sidelying positions and the fetal position are slightly less beneficial. Sitting requires adequate low back support, reclining attitude, and frequent change of position. Standing to perform simple self-care tasks is taught and practiced. Patients are encouraged to place one foot in a "barroom" position or to lean on hands or elbows to unload the spine. Sleeping positions are reviewed. The hook-lying or fetal position is encouraged.

If the patient is on a rest program prescribed by the physician, he returns home for a period of 1 week. If the patient works, day one continues with a review of protective body mechanics and work activities. The low intradiscal pressure theory applies to all work activities, and the pelvic tilt or abdominal tightening maneuver is taught as protection when moving about in the upright posture. Resting positions and first aid are taught for relief of job-related low back pain. The patient is then sent back to the working environment for 3 days' time and then returns to back school.

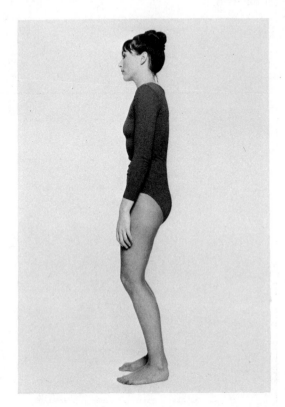

Fig. 4-15. Pelvic tilt. Back straight, stomach in, buttocks tucked under, and knees bent.
From Mulry, R.C., White, A.H., and Klein, E.A.: The portable back school: a home study program for proper back care, St. Louis, 1981, The C.V. Mosby Co.

DAY TWO

Day two continues with the theory that spinal pain is related to the position and motion of the lumbar spine. The resting positions of day one are reviewed for their application by giving a short verbal or written quiz. Household activities are evaluated (Fig. 4-16). A physical evaluation is performed on patients with continued complaints of sciatica or worsening symptoms. The boxed material on pp. 70 and 71 further defines the goals and schedule for day two.

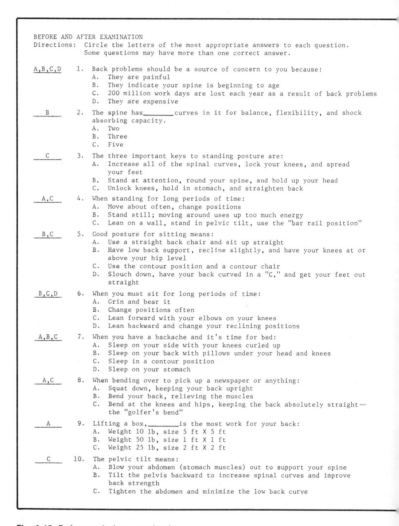

BEFORE AND AFTER EXAMINATION
Directions: Circle the letters of the most appropriate answers to each question. Some questions may have more than one correct answer.

A,B,C,D   1. Back problems should be a source of concern to you because:
       A. They are painful
       B. They indicate your spine is beginning to age
       C. 200 million work days are lost each year as a result of back problems
       D. They are expensive

B   2. The spine has_____curves in it for balance, flexibility, and shock absorbing capacity.
       A. Two
       B. Three
       C. Five

C   3. The three important keys to standing posture are:
       A. Increase all of the spinal curves, lock your knees, and spread your feet
       B. Stand at attention, round your spine, and hold up your head
       C. Unlock knees, hold in stomach, and straighten back

A,C   4. When standing for long periods of time:
       A. Move about often, change positions
       B. Stand still; moving around uses up too much energy
       C. Lean on a wall, stand in pelvic tilt, use the "bar rail position"

B,C   5. Good posture for sitting means:
       A. Use a straight back chair and sit up straight
       B. Have low back support, recline slightly, and have your knees at or above your hip level
       C. Use the contour position and a contour chair
       D. Slouch down, have your back curved in a "C," and get your feet out straight

B,C,D   6. When you must sit for long periods of time:
       A. Grin and bear it
       B. Change positions often
       C. Lean forward with your elbows on your knees
       D. Lean backward and change your reclining positions

A,B,C   7. When you have a backache and it's time for bed:
       A. Sleep on your side with your knees curled up
       B. Sleep on your back with pillows under your head and knees
       C. Sleep in a contour position
       D. Sleep on your stomach

A,C   8. When bending over to pick up a newspaper or anything:
       A. Squat down, keeping your back upright
       B. Bend your back, relieving the muscles
       C. Bend at the knees and hips, keeping the back absolutely straight— the "golfer's bend"

A   9. Lifting a box,_____is the most work for your back:
       A. Weight 10 lb, size 5 ft X 5 ft
       B. Weight 50 lb, size 1 ft X 1 ft
       C. Weight 25 lb, size 2 ft X 2 ft

C   10. The pelvic tilt means:
       A. Blow your abdomen (stomach muscles) out to support your spine
       B. Tilt the pelvis backward to increase spinal curves and improve back strength
       C. Tighten the abdomen and minimize the low back curve

Fig. 4-16. Before and after examination.

B	11.	For good balance when lifting: A. Keep your feet together and use your back B. Keep your feet wide apart, hold the load close, and use the pelvic tilt C. Keep your feet wide apart, sway your back, and get the load at chest height
A	12.	When reaching over, up, or out with any load: A. Use the pelvic tilt and keep your feet wide apart B. Sway your spine to get more height and distance C. Keep your feet together and use your arms to do the work
C	13.	Lifting should be done: A. Rapidly, as fast as you can, to get rid of that load B. With speed to get momentum C. Smoothly, with rhythm
B	14.	When playing any sport or doing any recreational activity the_____ will be your best back protection: A. Umpire B. Pelvic tilt (abdominal muscles) C. Sway back
B,C	15.	When twisting: A. Move around quickly to avoid strain B. Pivot around as one unit C. Use the pelvic tilt, setting your abdomen before you move
A,B,C	16.	Round-back bending and_____ will certainly strain and possibly injure your back: A. Lifting B. Twisting C. Reaching out for a load
A	17.	When lifting any load, this is the crucial factor: A. Keep it close to your body B. Use a machine C. Hold it at a distance from you to improve your balance and reach
D	18.	If you were to eliminate one motion from your daily life to protect your spine, it would be: A. Sitting B. Lifting C. Bending D. Twisting
B,C,D	19.	These muscles are the ones to consider when planning exercises for your back problems: A. Your vocal cords B. Your back muscles need to be strengthened C. Your stomach muscles need to be strengthened and your hamstring muscles stretched D. Your thigh muscles need to be strengthened
A	20.	These factors are the most important when it comes to back health care: A. Rest, exercise, body mechanics, and work task design B. Exercise and strong muscles C. Machines to do your work for you and a good doctor to keep you well

Day two Goals and schedule

GOALS

Therapist
Determine symptoms, recovery, progress
Assess day one instructions
Evaluate resting positions
Evaluate posture
Assess home activity problems and train in daily standing work/activities

Patient
Understand standing work positions
Know concept of protective body mechanics for resting, sitting, and standing work; bending, reaching, pushing, and pulling
Comprehend exercises, if given
Understand first aid measures for recurring or worsening pain

SCHEDULE

Time (minutes)	Goals	Methods	Materials presented	Evaluation
10 (20 with physical evaluation)	Determine patient problems with day one instructions; recovery	Interview, consult physical evaluation, if needed	Question and discussion of day one	Patient demonstration of correct posture, standing, sitting, lying down
10	Introduce standing working positions, reaching, lifting	AV lecture	Program with concepts of protective body work	Patient discussion and demonstration
10	Introduce concepts of protective body mechanics in everyday activities	AV program	Activities of daily living slides; additional presentations as necessary	Patient discussion

SCHEDULE—cont'd

Time (minutes)	Goals	Methods	Materials presented	Evaluation
20	Correct patient performance of protective body mechanics for standing, reaching, bending, lifting, pushing, pulling	Obstacle course training	Standing, reaching, straight spine bending, lifting techniques for light and heavy loads, pushing, pulling	Patient demonstration
15	Special needs; introduce lifting, office work, specific job-related activities	AV program and lecture	Specific job-related activities or activities of daily living needs	Patient discussion
20	Correct patient performance of special needs protective body mechanics	Obstacle course training	Specific job-related activities or activities of daily living mechanics required	Patient demonstration
15	Train patient in correct performance or exercise, if required	Demonstration of written order	Isometric exercises of pelvic tilt, partial sit-up, wall slide hold, straight leg raise stretch as ordered	Patient performance and discussion

Patient instruction

Pelvic tilt. Pelvic tilt is a protective maneuver for the lumbar spine (Fig. 4-15). The pelvis is tilted or tucked under the spine. This maneuver requires the use of abdominal, pelvic, and hip musculature pulling the hips and pelvis forward. It reduces the prominence of the buttocks, flattens the lumbar spine, and increases intraabdominal pressure. The pelvic tilt or abdominal compression routine is taught to reduce both segmental motion of the spine and loading pressures during moving activities, such as house cleaning, sweeping and vacuuming, mowing the lawn, or weeding the garden. The pelvic tilt maneuver is also taught as protection during reaching, twisting, returning from a squatting position, and as the correct rhythm in returning from bending-or stooping postures. The patient is instructed in light load handling, using the ergonomic concepts of shortening the distance from body to load, squatting to lift, and using the pelvic tilt to lessen the load on the spine, as well as the motion within the spine.

Bending body mechanics. The straight back or "golfer's" method of bending is included at this time to challenge the patient's coordination and theory application abilities. The patient is instructed to use this bend during waist-high work, such as brushing the teeth, washing the hair, placing dishes in the dishwasher, or using the refrigerator, oven, or stove. The pelvic tilt — abdominal compression maneuver is added to the straight back bend for all overextended work, such as laboring under the hood of the automobile, working at a workbench, or repairing the plumbing on a sink (Chapter 6).

Normal bending to reach to the ground from a standing position occurs first at the lumbar spine (Fig. 4-17, A). This requires a minimum of muscular use and expenditure of energy. The trunk is simply allowed to fall forward by the forces of gravity while the large strong paraspinal muscles allow the trunk to move forward until it totally rests the vertebral ligamentous structures. The paraspinal muscles then cease doing their job. This is a precarious position in that a small amount of further loading can do damage to any number of lumbar structures, but most notably the disc. In returning to the upright position from this type of bend, the paraspinal muscles reactivate and pull the trunk back to an erect position (Fig. 4-17, B).

A second type of bend uses mostly the hips (Fig. 4-17, C). The knees are relatively straight, and the back is straight. The trunk again is allowed to fall forward by the use of normal gravity but paraspinal muscles hold the lumbar spine straight so that the position of the vertebral segments remains the same as it is when erect. This does not allow the vertebral segments to position themselves in full flexion in such a way that there is danger to the disc and ligamentous structures. It does require considerable physical effort, both of the paraspinal muscles during the continual bend and of the muscles that cross the hip, which must be used to a great extent to hold the position and to pull the trunk back upright. Most difficult about this type of bending is the coordination. Humans are so used to bending from their backs and knees that they generally have a difficult time disconnecting the use of the lumbar spine and isolating use of the hips in this fashion. It is a necessary bend, however, for many activities, such as getting things out of the trunk of a car. To maintain this type of bend requires considerable abdominal muscular endurance.

The third type of bend and the one that is probably most universally safe and usable is

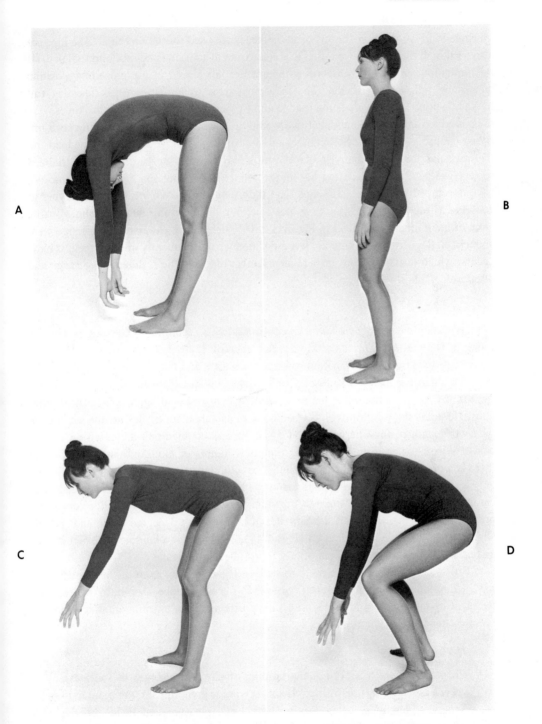

Fig. 4-17. Bending body mechanics. **A,** Lumbar back bend. **B,** Erect posture using pelvic tilt. **C,** Hip and straight back bend. **D,** Hip, knee, and back bend.
From Mulry, R.C., White, A.H., and Klein, E.A.: The portable back school: a home study program for proper back care, St. Louis, 1981, The C.V. Mosby Co.

illustrated in Fig. 4-17, *D*. In this bend the knees are used for the first time. The hips are also used, and the back is even used to some extent. The back is not allowed to flex to its full limitation so that the vertebral structures are not placed in the precarious position created by full lumbar flexion. The paraspinal muscles remain actively resisting full lumbar flexion. The hips are being used to almost their maximum extent. If the knees were to be used to their maximum extent, we would be creating a crouch or kneeling position. By proper use and coordination in this kind of a bend and lift, we are sharing the load and the muscular forces on many joints and muscles. Unfortunately, in our industrialized society, we have been overusing our lumbar spines in bending and lifting positions. We have developed weak legs, stiff hips, and tight hamstrings. We are by nature trying to conserve as much physical energy as possible. We therefore fall into the habit of using more of the lumbar spine bend in Fig. 4-17, *A*, which causes excessive long-range wear and tear on the vertebral segments. It is a position we are frequently in when the last blow occurs, which leads to a torn or herniated lumbar disc and the resultant long-range and often irreparable low back pain.

Exercises

All patients are taught a home exercise program to reinforce their body mechanics training. The partial sit-up is used to develop abdominal strengthening (Fig. 4-18). This exercise is done in a supine position with the knees bent and the feet flat on the floor. The patient tightens his abdominal muscles while raising his shoulders and shoulder blades off the surface. He does not crane his neck forward, which would aggravate cervical problems. He holds the position with his head, neck, and shoulder blades off the surface for whatever length of time he can tolerate. The time is counted and increased on a daily basis. We ask for an isometric holding time of 1 minute or more in this position unless there is a previous history of cardiovascular or vascular disease.

Isometric training is also applied to the quadriceps muscles unless there is a history of cardiovascular, vascular, or knee dysfunction. The human chair, wall slide, or skier's position against the wall with the hips flexed at a 60- to 90-degree angle and the feet slightly in front of the knees is used (Fig. 4-19). We look for a holding time of 1 minute as fair and 3 minutes as excellent ability to use these muscles.

Patients are encouraged to perform both of these training exercises at least twice a day, adding more holding time each session. In our experience, 3 minutes of isometric partal sit-up hold and 5 minutes of wall slide position are not uncommon after 1 month's faithful attendance to this routine.

The working patient

When the patient is working, the training of day two changes to some extent. A work- needs assessment is performed. If sitting work is predominant, the training is aimed at sedentary ergonomics, using the low intradiscal pressure and EMG theories. The concepts of chair design, function, and selection are emphasized. The patients are taught the fundamentals of chair adjustment and work environment ergonomics. The work situation is simulated and practiced on the obstacle course. This is as easily performed in groups as individually. As mentioned earlier, protective body mechanics concepts, such

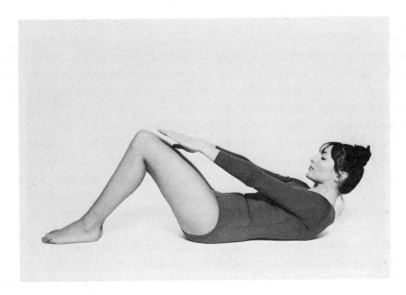

Fig. 4-18. Partial sit-up.
From Mulry, R.C., White, A.H., and Klein, E.A.: The portable back school: a home study program for proper back care, St. Louis, 1981, The C.V. Mosby Co.

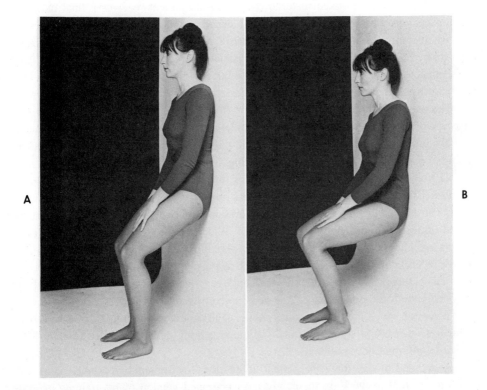

Fig. 4-19. A and **B.** Wall slide hold, human chair, or skier's position.
From Mulry, R.C., White, A.H., and Klein, E.A.: The portable back school: a home study program for proper back care, St. Louis, 1981, The C.V. Mosby Co.

as the pelvic tilt, straight back bend, and bending rhythm, are taught from seated as well as standing positions. More details are given in Chapter 7.

The exercise program for the sedentary worker is the same as that for the nonworking patient. We add to this a series of modified stretches done in the chair and seated isometric training exercises for the paravertebral extensors, especially the mid-scapular abductors. All exercises requiring seated lumbar flexion are eliminated.

When the nature of the work is predominately standing, the format closely follows that for the nonworking patient. Examples of work- and job-related situations are used in place of household activities. The mechanics of load handling and shifting are taught using the concepts of shortened distance between body and load, pelvic tilt, and avoidance of bending or stooped activity for any prolonged period of time. The exercise program includes isometric training for the abdominal and quadriceps musculature, adding to this isometric training for the trunk extensors and isotonic training for the leg muscles in aerobic activities. We encourage such activities as swimming, walking, or stationary bicycling. A warm-up program of leg stretches is taught before working activities; all stretches should be done in the static and protected positions. All patients return to back school in 1 week after doing the exercises presented.

DAY THREE

On day three (see boxed material on p. 77) the patient receives a final quiz and performs a final obstacle course to test his coordination and ability. He receives an exercise tolerance test of the wall slide and partial sit-up exercises. A physical evaluation is performed if deemed necessary by the physician.

Patients should receive instruction and practice on heavy lifting or cumbersome load handling, using the protective body mechanics concepts already introduced.

The patient still off work is instructed on the basics of body mechanics for his specific type of work. Instruction follows the guidelines of day two for the working patient.

The program is evaluated at this point. It may be considered a success, if the patient is able to control his pain in all of his working and resting positions.

The working patient is taught the basics of preventive body mechanics for sports activities. The same protective body mechanics rules may be used for all sports. Maximizing use of the pelvic tilt — abdominal compression maneuver protects the spine during weight lifting, twisting, and ballistic activites. Widening the narrow base of support and making maximum use of the knees will effect better motion translation into the legs. This is most helpful during ballistic activities, such as twisting, squash, racquetball, tennis, or American baseball. The basic rules are then applied to the sports needs of each patient and practiced either on the obstacle course or in a nearby park. Jogging and running are the most requested sports training activities we see. The patient is taught facts about footwear, warm-ups, stance and style, and finally protective body maneuvers. See Chapter 8 for additional information on athletes.

At the end of day three the patient is appraised of his remaining body mechanics deficiencies, told to work on them, given an upgraded version of his training exercise program, and sent back to the referring physician. The patient is scheduled for a recheck visit 1 month from the day-three visit.

Day three Goals and schedule

GOALS

Therapist
Determine recovery by physical evaluation
Assess performance of protective body mechanics on obstacle course
Evaluate understanding of key concepts in final examination
Train patient in protective body mechanics for sports and recreation

Patient
Understand the postural mechanism that causes the back-related pain
Demonstrate and understand the rationale for protective body mechanics during resting, standing,
    lying, sitting; working postures of standing, bending, lifting, reaching, pushing, pulling, and
    sitting; and recreational activities
Discuss and demonstrate first aid measures for low back pain
Discuss progression and performance of exercises, if given

SCHEDULE

Time (minutes)	Goals	Methods	Materials presented	Evaluation
5	Review progress	Interview	Days one and two	Therapist interview
15	Assess understanding of concepts of protective body mechanics	Written quiz	Standing, sitting, lying positioning, lifting and carrying, resting positions, exercise	Therapist grades quiz
10	Assess recovery by physical evaluation	Physical evaluation	Physical evaluation form	Therapist performs evaluation
5	Patient dresses			
30	Assess practical application of protective body mechanics	Obstacle	Obstable course form and simulated job situation, lifting situations	Therapist scores obstacle course form
10	Teach patient appropriate exercise	Therapist-patient demonstration	Specific isometric exercise	Patient demonstration
15	Specific problems	Discussion	Specific problems	Discussion

DAY FOUR

At the recheck visit (see boxed material below) the patient is again quizzed on the fundamentals presented, tested on the application on the obstacle course, tested on exercise proficiency, and progress is measured. This becomes a problem-solving day for the patient, allowing him to further evaluate ergonomic situations. If there is no further low back dysfunction or sciatica present, the exercise program is upgraded to include maximum stretch, strength, and self-mobilization exercises as maintenance. The patient is cautioned to balance all extensor training of trunk muscles with flexor training and activity. The patient is taught to use both the acute protective body mechanics of daily living and the first aid measures taught on day one, if a low back problem arises in the future.

Day four Goals and schedule

GOALS

Therapist
Perform physical evaluation
Assess understanding of key concepts by quizzing
Assist patient in problem-solving process
Evaluate performance of protective body mechanics on the obstacle course

Patient
Demonstrate and understand the rationale for protective body mechanics during resting, recreation, and while working.
Discuss and begin problem solving for special situations

SCHEDULE

Time (minutes)	Goals	Methods	Materials presented	Evaluation
10	Quiz, review progress	Quiz, interview	Quiz days one through three	Quiz, interview
15	Assess physical evaluation	Physical evaluation	Physical evaluation	Physical
20	Assess practical application of protective body mechanics	Obstacle course	Obstacle course	Evaluation, therapist scores obstacle course interview
15	Problem solving specific areas	Interview, discussion	Patient problems	Interview

• • •

The material presented in this chapter up to this point represents the basic back school format as it developed in San Francisco at the California Back School. It has been greatly successful in helping orthopaedic surgeons and hospitals to treat their back pain patients more effectively. We realize it is not possible for physicians in many communities to develop such an extensive program. We have therefore developed a smaller and easy-to-institute back school program. We have taken the basic information and condensed it into two small booklets and a few audiovisual programs. This can be instituted by any physician's office with minimal paramedical assistance.

VARIATIONS ON THE BASIC BACK SCHOOL

All patients do not become totally pain free and in control of their conditions with a standard outpatient back school. There may be several reasons for this. The patient may have a physical condition, such as spinal stenosis or a herniated disc that is beyond the capabilities of control by simple back education and body mechanics. That individual needs more intensive care, probably in a hospital situation where total rest and diagnostic and therapeutic procedures can be performed to help him attain a comfortable, pain-free state. This might even require surgery eventually. The back school assists in all hospital evaluation, treatment, and explanation.

Another reason for a patient not improving might be because a great part of his problem is psychogenic. He may be unconsciously magnifying or aggravating his condition. This at times can be dealt with as an outpatient in the back school. More often, however, the back pain is such a complex combination of physical, emotional, and environmental problems that it is best to have the patient in the hospital in a pain ward or rehabilitation ward setting. Here the back school interdigitates with a psychologist and others (multidisciplinary team) who use behavioral modification in an operant conditioning type of atmosphere. This back school training is more sophisticated and is explained later.

A third reason for failure of the basic outpatient back school is the possibility that the requirements of the patient and his environment are greater than the capabilities of his body with his current disease. For instance the patient may want to engage in some heavy athletics or he may have a job that is impossible to perform, considering his current level of conditioning and his disease state. Therefore he has to either alter his environment or his body. This kind of conditioning may require a sports medicine center to strengthen the appropriate musculature and aid him in changing his techniques of body mechanics for the individual tasks. This may mean relearning to perform a certain sport.

The last variety of back school is the industrial back school. Here the back school instructor is mainly concerned with ergonomics. Through ergonomics the patient's job is altered to fit a normal working back and may even be altered to suit a diseased back. Motivation factors are also extremely important in the industrial patient. The back school instructor can learn a great deal about a patient's motivation as the job is discussed and demonstrated. The work situation is simulated and practiced on the obstacle course.

THE PSYCHOLOGICAL ENVIRONMENT

There is no physical illness known to man that does not have psychological impact. For some reason low back pain has more psychological overtones than most other physical illnesses. This may partially be the result of learned behavior. We have seen during our lives many people who have been crippled from back pain. We see, hear, and read much about back pain and have fears about it. Back pain does things to our bodies that we do not understand. A person can be bent over and unable to straighten up and yet cannot see an understandable cause. When a person has an infection, he understands from general education something about the mechanism of bacteria and inflammation. We do not have any general education about back pain and its causes.

Many physicians believe that the psychological state is responsible for much, if not all, of the back pain. We know that tension and pressure can produce headaches. It is quite probable that tension and pressure can cause, if not greatly aggravate, backache. We have found that techniques such as biofeedback, hypnosis, relaxation therapy, and muscle relaxants can relieve backache. As we take their histories, most patients volunteer the information that they notice that their back pain gets worse when they are upset, angry, or otherwise under emotional tension.

Back pain frequently interferes and sometimes totally destroys a person's social and emotional environment. Because of constant complaining and poor response to all treatment, family and friends frequently turn away. There is nothing to see that explains to other people why the patient is incapacitated. He does not have a cast or a sling, an eye patch, or a cane to indicate to others that he is truly sick.

We must remember also that pain is a learned response. We all learn how to interpret and express pain differently. Animals can be taught to not only accept, but look forward to what we would ordinarily consider painful stimuli. A slight discomfort for one person can be interpreted by another person as an excrutiating pain. This difference in the experience of pain makes it an impossible task for the physician to know how to treat a particular person. It takes a great amount of time living with an individual and seeing him under many circumstances to know how he responds to pain. This is part of the reason that surgery for low back pain has such a bad reputation. Despite surgery, the aging process continues producing local inflammation. If the afflicted individual interprets this as excrutiating pain, he will have many years of invalidism, whereas another individual suffering the same condition accepts the discomfort as a little arthritis or "growing-old pains."

We are sometimes able to alter a person's psychological outlook toward his back pain. He can be educated as to the cause of his pain and when he understands this, the pain is easier to accept. Pain behavior can be modified much as we modify the behavior of a growing child. This is called behavioral modification. If a pain patient is given verbal and other rewards for accepting his pain and going on with productive activities, he becomes less aware of his pain. In a similar way he can be given verbal and environmental punishments for "overreacting" to his pain.

Some pain patients are psychologically ill. They have an unconscious need to have pain. It may represent a punishment for some unconscious guilt. People with such deep-seated psychological problems need professional psychiatric care. People with minor psychological problems are more frequently encountered. Perhaps these forms should not even be called illness. There is a conscious or unconscious attempt on these people's part to control their environments by the pain that they have. This can be in the form of getting attention that would not be given without the pain. Many an inattentive wife has been kept at home soothing her husband's aching back. Back pain is used by many to avoid physically or psychologically uncomfortable situations. A man may use his pain to avoid going to a job that is physically or psychologically too strenuous for him. Pain is used around the home to escape chores, housework, and sexual activities. All of these are learned behaviors and can be easily identified and altered without the need for extensive psychiatric involvement.

All back schools use some psychological techniques. The ultimate is the operant conditioning program found in most spinal centers. The original and most advanced operant conditioning program, to my knowledge, is that of Dr. Fordyce in Seattle, Washington. This is a pain control program that is based on the concepts of behavioral modification. It is essentially an inhouse program that takes several weeks to several months. It involves detoxification of patients who are addicted, intensive psychological studies, and subsequent psychological recycling of the patient's attitude toward his pain. There must also be adjustments in the attitude of the patient's family; environmental changes are necessary if either of these factors contribute to the patient's pain. This type of program requires at least one well-trained psychologist. It is generally felt that one psychologist can handle as many as four patients undergoing one of these programs. At the same time that the psychological environment and drug environment are being controlled, the patient undergoes a physical therapy program that gradually advances him from below his usual functioning level to a maximum physical functioning level. He receives verbal and other psychological rewards as he advances. These programs require a team of experts in behavioral modification, all of whom are helping the patient over the emotional hurdles and stimulating him in the right direction to a home environment that may have been keeping the patient psychologically disabled. These types of programs generally will not accept a patient, if there is any further hope of a cure by surgery or other medical means.

Most other back training programs, whether they are inpatient or outpatient, use the basic concept of behavioral modification in some form. The group education back programs have a built-in psychological stimulus for the patient. There are other patients present who are improving and are enthusiastic. They give each other rewards much as Alcoholics Anonymous and Weight Watchers. The lecturers of group programs should be well aware of the behavioral modification techniques so that they can guide their groups as a whole, or stimulate certain individuals who are falling behind. In the individualized back school programs where one therapist works with one patient, these "functional" patients are frequently the most resistant to treatment and need special behavioral modification techniques. We frequently use a psychologist in the back school to help us with these resistant individuals. There are very few outpatient operant conditioning programs. When we fail with outpatients because of psychological problems, we recommend admission to an inpatient operant conditioning program.

5 HOSPITAL BACK SCHOOL

Hospital back school can be composed of as many as four different programs, depending on the needs of the community and the availability of support personnel. The four broad categories are (1) inpatient acute conservative care, (2) inpatient before and after surgical care, (3) inpatient pain rehabilitation, and (4) extended day care hospital program. Fig. 5-1 demonstrates the flow between these programs. Each program is discussed in detail as to its philosophy, aim, and requirements.

A new patient who finds himself in the emergency room or cast room with very disabling back or leg pain may not be able to go home for outpatient care and back school. An epidural block is frequently done in the acute phase in an attempt to get the patient home and to manage his condition as an outpatient. In cases when the patient's condition is too severe or the patient's home environment is totally nonsupportive, the patient is put in the inpatient acute conservative care program. This might mean 1 to 5 days of bed rest, medication, blocks, modalities, education, and training so that the patient can then be discharged with a follow-up done by the outpatient back school.

If this patient does not improve in a few days, he becomes part of the inpatient before and after surgical care program. This includes diagnostic measures, an explanation of procedures and philosophy of surgical approaches, preparation for surgery, and a follow-up after surgery, if it is performed.

The inpatient pain management and rehabilitation program is mainly for patients who cannot have any further surgical procedures but they do have chronic low back pain that requires extensive training and a psychological push to overcome pain behavior and deeply ingrained bad habits. These patients are too complicated and resistive to outpatient conservative measures to have success in an outpatient back school setting. Occasionally one of these patients requires further surgery. In that case he is transferred to the before and after surgical inpatient program but is still supported before and after the surgery by the pain rehabilitation program.

After discharge from the hospital and the pain rehabilitation program, many patients are still in need of long-range outpatient support and encouragement. This is more than the normal outpatient back school setting can provide. Therefore these patients are seen in the extended hospital day care program, where they can have the 8 hours a day of support and pain control that the inpatient programs provide, but these patients are not in need of staying in the hospital overnight. Some patients can be placed in this program without ever having to be admitted to the hospital. Following is a discussion of each one of these areas in greater detail.

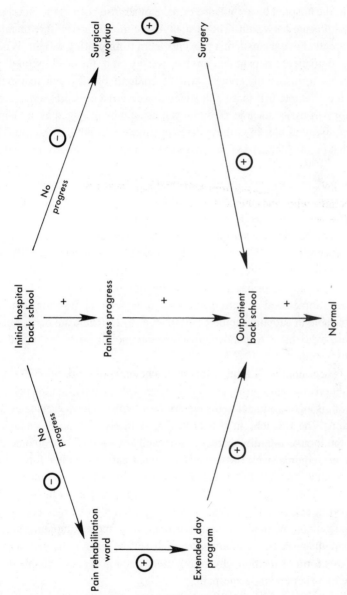

Fig. 5-1. Program flow

INPATIENT ACUTE CONSERVATIVE CARE PROGRAM

The inpatient acute conservative care program usually involves diagnostic categories such as acutely herniated lumbar discs with or without neurological deficit, spinal stenosis, spondylolisthesis, and fracture. These individuals in these categories have either been brought to the hospital by ambulance or have otherwise been in the emergency room or cast room with acute back pain. They usually have muscle spasm, are unable to stand erect, and frequently have leg pain that prevents them from bearing weight. When seen as an emergency outpatient, depending on the facility and the back school personnel available, various forms of injections, such as epidural blocks, and manipulations or mobilizations are attempted. If these outpatient conservative measures are successful and the patient improves by as much as 50%, he can usually be managed as an outpatient. In our experience, epidural blocks in these cases are successful 80% of the time. Mobilization, such as that on the McKenzie form, works very well on the anulus tear and acute disc injuries.

When the patient does not improve sufficiently to be managed as an outpatient, he is placed in the inpatient acute conservative care ward. Patients in the acute conservative care ward are generally confined to bed rest initially. It is necessary to find the position of maximum comfort. The back school is responsible for helping the patient determine what position is most comfortable. This is partially decided by the dynamic evaluation examination that is given to find what positions are most aggravating and most relieving. It is also found on a trial and error basis. Usually patients find that they are comfortable in a contour position. Some need an extreme contour or a jackknife position, whereas others are only comfortable in a totally supine position (Fig. 5-2). There are occasional patients, especially those who have responded to extension mobilization, who find the prone position is most comfortable (Fig. 5-3).

Traction is occasionally helpful to maintain a better contour position during bed rest. Having the traction apparatus arranged so that there is vertical pull on the pelvis, creating pelvic tilt in bed, is a good adjunct to the electric bed, which allows varying degrees of the contour position. The traction, in bed however, is rarely significant enough to create distraction of the lumbar interdiscal spaces. It is well known that to overcome the friction of the bed alone requires over 100 pounds for most patients. Other forms of traction, however, are possible and helpful. There are various forms of gravity lumbar traction that can be used with a Circ-O-Lectric bed or a Nelson bed. The patient lies in bed in gravity traction at varying degrees of tilt and for varying amounts of time, depending on the tolerance of the patient. We find that female patients have more complaints because of the pressure around their breasts. Mobilizations and self-mobilizations can be done while suspended in this form of traction. Inverted gravity traction is also valuable but harder to use with patients experiencing acute pain.

Various modalities can be applied at bed rest to assist in the patient's comfort. These include massage, ice massage, local heat in the form of K-pads or other heating devices, transcutaneous stimulators, biofeedback, and neuroprobe. These can all be used by the therapist, depending on the patient's tolerance, needs, and the particular philosophy of the back school therapist.

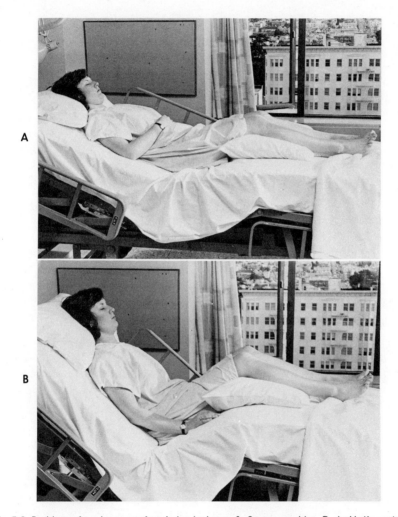

Fig. 5-2. Positions of maximum comfort during bed rest. **A,** Contour position, **B,** Jackknife position.

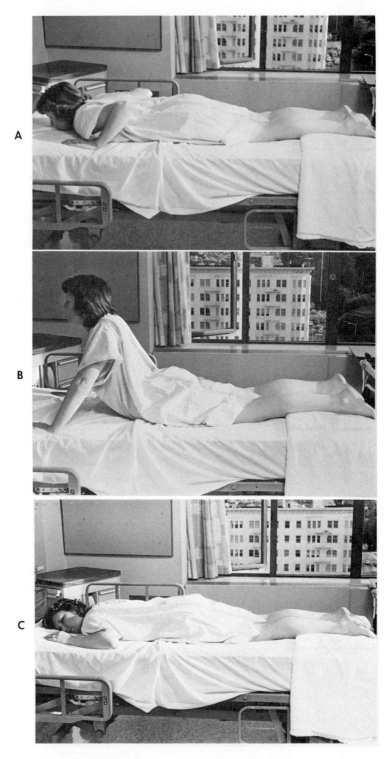

Fig. 5-3. Extension mobilization. **A,** Begin press-up position. **B,** Full press-up position (pelvis on bed and arms fully extended). **C,** Position of comfort for the patient who responds well to extension mobilization.

At times it is necessary to spend several days at complete bed rest. Fractures and acute herniated discs with neurological deficit may require a delicate balance between activity, position, and further damage. This can require log rolling, tilting beds, and at times what we call the "holey mattress." The holey mattress is a several-inch-thick piece of foam rubber mattress that is placed on the hospital bed. There is a hole approximately 1 foot square cut out for the use of a bedpan. The patient can be log rolled, the plug of foam rubber removed from the hole, and a bedpan placed under him (Fig. 5-4). The patient is then log rolled back over the hole and allowed to use the bedpan, thus not having to arch the back or change position significantly, which helps in causing no further damage to the spine. At times a patient's condition is so acute that he requires as long as 1 or 2 weeks on this type of a mattress. Unstable fractures can be managed for months in this fashion. We

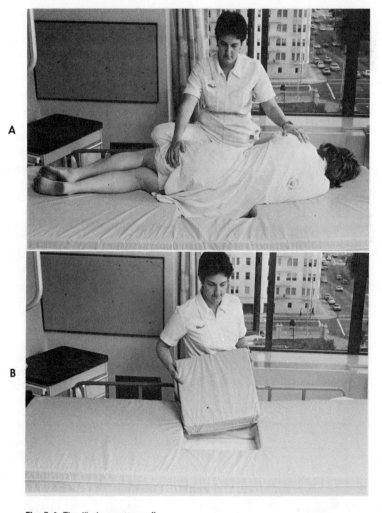

Fig. 5-4. The "holey mattress."

Table 5-1. Progressive bed exercise routine

Exercise	Position	Cues	Purpose
Abdominal sets	Contour	Push back into bed Tighten abdomen	Preparation for log rolling
Gluteal sets	Contour	Pinch buttocks together	Preparation for log rolling
Deep breathing with upper extremity ROM	Contour	Arms out with inhalation Arms in with exhalation	Concentration on deep breathing Relaxation Maintenance of upper extremity ROM Protection against atelectasis or pneumonia
Ankle circles	Contour	Move ankle slowly in directions; circle one way and then the opposite	Maintenance of ankle ROM Protection against phlebitis with exercises
Isometric triceps	Contour	Push elbows into bed	Preparation for elbow bend technique Maintenance of strength
Pelvic tilt	Contour	Combination of gluteal and abdominal sets	Preparation for ambulation and good body mechanics
Quadriceps sets	One knee bent Exercise leg straight	Tighten thigh muscles	Maintenance of lower extremity strength Key to lifting body mechanics
Straight leg raise	One knee bent Exercise leg straight	Tighten thigh— breathe in; lift leg —breathe out; tighten—breathe in; lower leg— —breathe out	Straight leg raise activity indicates when patient is ready to get out of bed

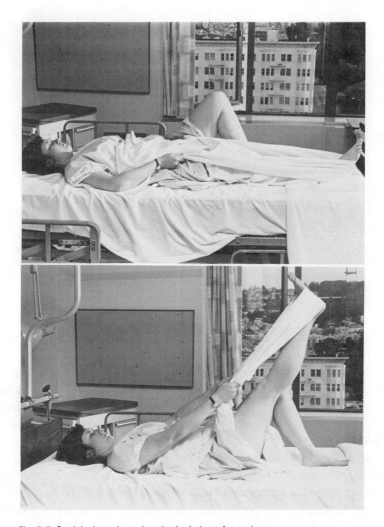

Fig. 5-5. Straight leg raise using the bed sheet for assistance.

are mainly dealing, however, with shorter term diseases of disc and nerve root involvement. Our aim is to get the inflammation to subside as rapidly as possible with the use of oral or injectable cortisone along with maximum rest and then get the patient moving as rapidly as possible with whatever support, body mechanics, or assistance necessary.

When the patient is comfortable at bed rest, we begin painless increases in activity (Table 5-1) (Figs. 5-5 and 5-6). At bed rest most patients can be doing isometric tightening of their abdominal muscles and quadriceps muscles. They can be using light weights for their upper extremities. They are allowed to change their positions as long as they remain painless. They can increase the contour position of the bed until they are reclining. They are assisted in log rolling and changing positions and the degree of straight

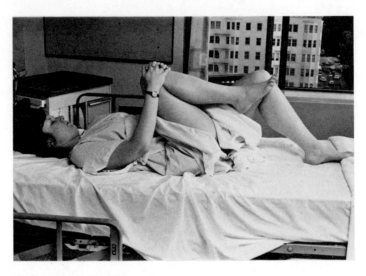

Fig. 5-6. Knee-to-chest exercise.

leg raising, muscle spasm, and motion is tested daily, taking care not to create any great amount of pain. They are tested, for instance, in straight leg raising until there is just slight discomfort and then they are observed to be sure it does not cause any long-range recurrence of pain. We try to keep analgesics, sedatives, tranquilizers, and other medications to a minimum because they can confuse the pain picture and make it difficult for the back school therapist, as well as the patient, to know the current state of inflammation and activity level.

When it is possible to do so painlessly, the patient moves from the bed rest position to standing. Minimal time is spent sitting and then only in a very erect upright position (Fig. 5-7). A Nelson bed or tilt table is sometimes necessary to get the patient on his feet. The patient learns pelvic tilt positioning, abdominal tightening, and use of the knees in bed, to keep his spine in the most comfortable position. As he achieves an erect position, he learns to maintain the same immobilization techniques to keep the spine in the most appropriate position for comfort (Fig 5-8). Most of the time this represents a neutral position, which is achieved by pelvic tilt, partial knee flexion, and abdominal tightening. This is not a flexion position but a neutral position. If extension is the most appropriate position, he learns to sit and stand in a hyperlordotic or lumbar extension position. There are a few conditions that are better in actual lumbar flexion but, if that is the case, he is allowed to do so as long as it is the pain-free position.

If the patient is able to stand painlessly for several minutes, he can begin to ambulate. He may need a walker, crutches, cane, body jacket, or other supportive device to help him maintain a painless position as he increases activities. The time out of bed at first is only a matter of minutes. He then goes back to bed in the most comfortable position to be sure he does not have any relapse of the pain. If he has a relapse, further bed rest time is necessary and then attempts with other methods can be used to try to increase activity. If the activity

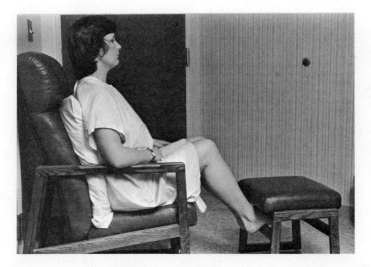

Fig. 5-7. Proper body mechanics for the bad back patient to use in sitting.

is well tolerated, the patient can ambulate in the same fashion again for longer periods of time with a few hours of bed rest between attempts. He is gradually allowed to ambulate independently. As rapidly as possible, the patient increases his activities to many laps around the ward and a few flights of stairs.

Considerable assistance and information need to be transferred from the back school therapist to the patient. During bed rest, the patient learns the basics of the working diagnosis in as simple a form as is necessary for him to understand enough to prevent future episodes of back pain. He needs to have a working knowledge of the body mechanics of his own condition and how to get back to safe activities. The patient sees pictures and audiovisual presentation regarding pelvic tilt, general back health care, and protective body mechanics. Procedures such as epidural blocks or facet blocks and diagnostic procedures such as myelograms and CT scans are explained to the patient by a back school therapist. The basic capabilities of the patient and the pain-producing and pain relieving activities are recorded and placed on a graph so that after procedures such as epidural blocks, the patient can score his pain and activity levels. The therapist can further evaluate the patient for determination of the success or failure of the blocks.

The therapist should have a very good working knowledge of corsets and flexion body jackets. In our setting the therapist is allowed to order the corset or body jacket, oversee the fitting of them, and take responsibility for getting the patient accustomed to them as the patient's activity is increased and he is discharged from the hospital. The back school therapist generally is in charge of the gravity lumbar traction, pool therapy, and modalities. The physician takes charge of the medication control with advice from the therapist. The physician does the epidural block at his own recommendation but also frequently does one at the recommendation of the back school therapist.

As the patient improves and is able to ambulate without pain, further exercises are

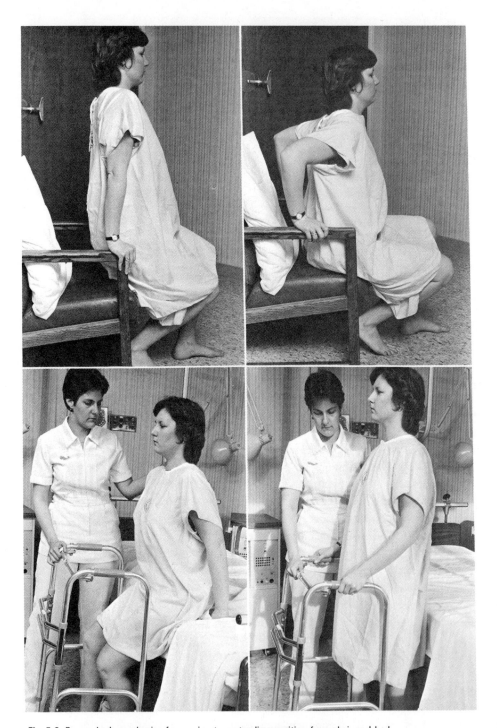

Fig. 5-8. Proper body mechanics for coming to a standing position from chair and bed.

given depending on his condition and ability. He can go to a sports medicine center and begin receiving instruction on working out with Nautilus and Cybex equipment. He can (with equal value) go to the physical therapy department and use wall pulley exercises, pool therapy, and other forms of active-resistive exercises. He eventually uses the acquired strength for learning and using proper body mechanics to remain pain free and avoid future injuries. As soon as the patient's pain subsides adequately to allow him to return to his home environment requirements, he is discharged and returns for a follow-up to the outpatient back school. If the patient is in the category of a pain and rehabilitation patient, he can be transferred to the inpatient pain rehabilitation ward. If he is not so severe a psychosocial rehabilitation problem that he needs the inpatient program, he can be discharged from the conservative care program and be returned to the extended day care program for outpatient pain rehabilitation.

THE BEFORE AND AFTER SURGICAL HOSPITAL PROGRAM

The inpatient with acute pain who does not improve with conservative measures and who is deemed a potential surgical candidate becomes a part of a program that is aimed toward surgery (the before and after surgical hospital program). He must undergo certain diagnostic tests that can overlap into the conservative care program. The back school physical therapist explains the procedures to be performed for diagnostic purposes. The blocks that have been performed therapeutically can also be done diagnostically. The patient receives information throughout the hospital course with regard to the likelihood of needing surgery, the time factors, and the potential advantage to surgery over conservative care. Each procedure performed, including the myelogram, venogram, CT scan, EMG, diagnostic blocks, bone biopsy, disogram, and bone scan, is explained to the patient before it is done, and then the results are given to the patient by the back school physical therapist. The physician follows up this explanation with his conclusions and helps support the data given by the therapist. The ultimate decision for surgery is up to the patient and is finally decided on with a conference between the physician and the patient.

If surgery is decided on by the patient, the back school therapist helps prepare the patient by getting him in as good a physical condition as possible before surgery. Anticipated results and potential complications are described to the patient by the surgeon and the back school therapist. The patient is also told what is to be expected of him after surgery. He may receive postoperative transcutaneous stimulation. The use of drains, postoperative braces, bed rest, exercises, and activity level are all made clear to the patient before surgery.

Following surgery, the therapist applies transcutaneous stimulators as necessary. He begins ambulating the patient when indicated. He may even be responsible for removing drains and sutures. In the more precarious postoperative cases, the back school therapist may need to use a tilting table or Nelson bed in order to begin ambulating the patient. Some patients need postoperative bracing. If the patient is going to require more than a week of postoperative care, it is better to transfer him to the pain rehabilitation ward, where more constant attention from more than one physical therapist is available.

When the postoperative patient reaches a level of independence that is commensurate with his requirements at home, he can be discharged. It usually means that the patient is able to ambulate for several hundred yards, and handle several flights of stairs. If he is very infirm but has maximum support at home, the patient can be discharged with the use of a walker, crutches, or a cane. If the patient is doing very well in his postoperative course, he may go to a sports medicine center and begin heavier training activity before his discharge from the hospital.

At the time of discharge of a patient who had surgery, written and verbal instructions are given as to exactly what is expected of him for the first month. Each patient is supposed to do a certain amount of exercise and ambulation each day. He is to report to the back school, preferably to see the same back school physical therapist who helped him in the hospital before and after surgery.

This brings up the concept of the physical therapist/patient manager. Who is the ideal patient manager? The orthopaedic surgeon is mainly trained in surgical technique. Our medical-economic system cannot support a surgeon giving education and manipulation. The general practitioner and internist is not usually trained in back problems. The physiatrist, although he understands back problems quite well, does not have the time to do full dynamic evaluations, give mobilization exercises, teach back school, do EMGs, and deal with the minute-to-minute problems of the back patient. The physical therapist is the ideal individual to be a patient manager. He is trained in modalities, mobilization, manipulation, activities of daily living, and job-related activities. He has the time and receives adequate compensation under our current system to teach, give exercises, evaluate, mobilize, and otherwise manage low back pain patients.

PAIN REHABILITATION INPATIENT PROGRAM

Our fast-moving industrialized society is producing problems for its inhabitants. Our lack of exercise and training does not prepare us for what would otherwise be considered the normal tasks of living. The tasks imposed on our workers are inconceivable under the circumstances. Lifting 100-pound sacks at three per minute for 20 years is unfathomable. Allowances are not made in industry for a person to do heavy labor for 5 or 10 years and then transfer into lighter work in his older years. We have set outselves up for major problems because we lack the training, and we have become weaker from a combination of overeating and insufficient physical exercise. Employees are given rewards for not returning to work. They are paid to be on disability. In many cases, they can make more money being off work than they can working. Pain behavior is becoming more and more deeply ingrained in many members of our society. It seems to be giving some individuals a kind of attention or fulfillment that they cannot otherwise achieve.

For all of the previously mentioned reasons, physicians have found it necessary to develop pain rehabilitation wards that try to break down some of the pain patterns that have developed in our culture. This is not to say that there is no underlying physical cause for the patient's pain. His pain behavior and social circumstances, however, make recovery almost impossible by conventional medical means. It is possible to take a patient with psychosocial problems and control his total environment for many days or weeks. We can break down some of the adverse developing patterns and train him to accept his physical plight and display his pain patterns in a different way. This is the function of the inpatient pain rehabilitation program.

There are many forms of such inpatient programs. They range from strict behavioral modification with a psychologist for a minimum of 6 weeks to an industrial evaluation program that identifies the psychosocial components of the problem but does not even try to treat them.

The therapist in these types of programs does an evaluation, putting the patient through a variety of exercises and obstacle course activities. The patient's baseline ability level is identified. A program is then set up to progressively increase that baseline level of activity with rewards for activity but not for lack of activity. The patient takes responsibility for his own pain and activity and medication levels. Bed rest and medication are discouraged. Activity, strengthening, and proper back health care are strongly encouraged. It is well understood that when a patient enters such a program that surgery is not a possibility. If the patient feels that surgery is going to save him, or some other major procedure can be done to take the pain away, he is less likely to take the responsibility and try to control the pain problems. Families come in for family counseling. Everyone possible in the patient's environment needs to participate in encouraging him to overcome his psychosocial problems.

The basic back school principles permeate the rehabilitation pain program. The major underlying message is that the patient's pain is totally controllable and livable, if the patient is willing to develop adequate strength, use proper body mechanics, and train just as any athlete trains. This means that the patient needs to train through his pain, continuing exercises and not elaborating or dwelling on the pain. Even though there is an underlying physical condition that creates pain, the patient is able to be much more active and live a relatively normal existence with the same level of pain. He has been in a downhill spiral for many years, being less active because of the pain. He has gained weight and lost strength and therefore has been less active. He has basically become sedentary and has dwelled on the pain so much that he has no activity level; only total pain behavior. By reversing this downhill spiral, he is able to do normal activities and stop the pain behavior that is influencing everyone around him and giving no significant value to his life.

EXTENDED DAY CARE HOSPITAL PROGRAM

Patients who do not need as much 24-hour per day environmental control can sometimes be handled adequately as outpatients in an extended day care hospital program. They come to the hospital at 8:00 AM. and leave at 5:00 PM. During that period of time they receive all of the activities and guidance that the inpatients on the pain rehabilitation program receive. They may spend more time in the gymnasium or sports medicine facility. They may receive less psychological counseling or group therapy. This type of program is, of course, much less expensive and in my opinion is going to be the major program of the future. We cannot as a society take on all of the social and cultural ills and try to cure them in hospitals with the expense incurred by conventional hospital programs. Several programs have been developed around the country that use motel rooms, convalescent hospitals, and less extensive forms of housing for patients who are undergoing these programs. There is great value in these patients living and working together. They see themselves more objectively by observing other patients and learning from their mistakes, seeing people who are worse off, getting caught up in the enthusiasm of the group, and finding that they are improving despite themselves.

Once a patient accepts responsibility for his own pain and exercises and improves on his own, he can be discharged from the extended day program to an outpatient back school program that simply evaluates him once every week and then once every month until he is totally on his own. If a more extensive evaluation or bigger push in therapy is necessary, the patient can come back once a month to the outpatient extended care program for a 1-day evaluation during which each of the therapists who had previously been treating the patient takes him through the exercises, endurance, and various training programs to assess his progress and stimulate him to greater heights during the following month.

A typical day in an extended day care program or inpatient pain rehabilitation program consists of something like the following:

8:00 to 9:00 AM: General exercise program in a sports medicine center with gentle stretching exercises, followed by isometric exercises, and then use of the Nautilus equipment or wall pulleys to the extent that the particular patient is allowed.

9:00 to 10:00 AM: Back school education in the same setting, where a general lecture is given to all of the individuals regarding particular aspects of their lives; for example, lifting, housework, activities of daily living, and job-related activities.

10:00 to 11:00 AM: Relaxation therapy program.

11:00 AM to 12:00 PM: Group therapy.

12:00 to 1:00 PM: Patients eat together in a common area where proper body mechanics, good chairs, and general supervision is available for cooking, eating, and other kitchen and dining area activities.

1:00 to 2:00 PM: Individuals have single therapy sessions with their psychologists, counselors, or family members.

2:00 to 3:00 PM: Specific modalities are used in the form of biofeedback, transcutaneous stimulation, mobilization, and hanging traction.

3:00 to 4:00 PM: Entire group goes to the pool for exercise and training depending on each individual's level of activity.

3:00 to 4:00 PM: Endurance training in groups. This includes long walks or bicycling (stationary or in the park). Patients who are able to jog go with a therapist who can teach this activity safely and extensively.

4:00 to 5:00 PM: Patients see their physicians or other counselors, if they are going home, to be sure that home environmental problems have been solved and that there are no problems with transportation, family emotions, or other things that might sabotage the patient's progress before the next day. Other patients have a general lecture or audiovisual program on topics such as ergonomics, diet, well-being, or other things that will hopefully keep them motivated and give them something to think about or work on until the following day when they resume the program.

GENERAL CONSIDERATIONS FOR ALL HOSPITAL PROGRAMS

There is certain information that is common to all hospital programs, which is different from other back school programs. The basic back school aim of strengthening, educating and teaching proper body mechanics naturally applies to the inpatient program as well. Hospitalization generally implies the requirement of beds, gurneys, and wheelchairs. This is not necessarily true in the rehabilitation wards where the patients are generally using only the beds and then only at night. The inpatient situation, however, is a means of controlling the environment 24 hours per day. All the other hospital programs imply that the patient is going to need major assistance in becoming pain free, transferring for diagnostic tests, being cared for before and after surgery, and in general requiring acute medical care.

There is specialized information necessary for the patient and for all hospital personnel who are dealing with back patients. This information is not so important for the general care of patients who are having their tonsils removed or who have various broken bones, obstetric problems, etc. The following information (patient handling manual), however, is valuable for all hospital personnel for the safety and control of their own backs. The back school needs to oversee the hospital personnel to be sure that they are treating their patients' backs properly, as well as their own.

The basic principle behind patient handling for both the patient and hospital personnel is to keep the spine in a protected, painless position at all times. In the initial acute hospitalization we see that the patient is placed in a painless position. Great effort is expended by the patient and therapist to find a painless position by dynamic evaluation and trials of various positions. By applying knowledge of the diagnosis, biomechanics, anatomy, and simple observation, we are able to find the appropriate position for each patient. Rarely is a patient comfortable only in a sitting position. Mostly patients seek some form of reclining contour position. Most patients who have herniated discs feel worse in a sitting position, which makes transfer from department to department in a wheelchair unreasonable. Roughly transferring patients from gurney to bed or having patients force themselves onto bedpans can be quite detrimental to their major spinal problems. With such lack of consideration, any healing that occurred by proper positioning and rest is rapidly lost. The lack of knowledge by most hospital personnel in these principles makes it necessary to include the following patient handling manual.

Most of the information in the patient handling manual is aimed at the hospital personnel for techniques of transferring the patients so that they are not hurt. There is, however, a certain amount of information that the patients need to know. The back school instructor should make it very clear to the patient that he is the primary person responsible for protection of his back. Even if an unknowledgeable hospital employee tells him to jump out of bed and into a wheelchair, he naturally should not do so. It is amazing to see the number of patients who are willing to shirk the responsibility for their own backs by doing things that they know are going to be painful, simply because they were told to do something by a person in a white uniform. The early instruction by the back school hospital therapist is along this line. Find your pain-free position. Transfer from one position to another as long as you remain without pain. This almost always entails a pelvic tilt and tightening of the abdomen. Isometric abdominal exercises are started very early in the hospital course. Log rolling with the abdominal muscles tightened is an integral part of postoperative care. Techniques for getting in and out of bed are going to be used by the patients for the rest of their lives. Any activity or position that reproduces or increases the patients' pain is potentially dangerous, no matter who tells them to do so. There is always another way to accomplish the task and do it painlessly. This is dependent on strength, knowledge, and body mechanics.

APPENDIX

Patient handling manual

I. Moving patients in bed
   A. Basic body mechanics
      1. Elevate the bed to waist height.
      2. Move a patient one segment at a time, that is, feet, buttocks, shoulders, and head, if at all possible.
      3. Get help when needed.
      4. When moving patients up in bed, always turn your foot that is closest to the head of the bed in that direction.
      5. Your protective body mechanics involve keeping knees slightly bent, using pelvic tilt, keeping back as straight as possible, and rocking forward onto the lead foot instead of jerking or using the spine for all of the lifting or pulling movement.
   B. Turning patients in bed
      1. If possible, turn patients away from you, not toward you.
      2. Begin by crossing the patient's arms over his chest and bending up both knees.
      3. Push on the knees and the shoulder girdle at the same time, turning the patient away from you.
      4. During this pushing maneuver you should keep your knees bent, practice pelvic tilt, have your back as straight as possible.
   C. Moving patients up in bed with two assistants
      1. Use a draw sheet whenever possible.
      2. Use help whenever possible. Do not attempt to move a patient in a bed with a draw sheet alone.
      3. Ask the patient to help by pulling on the trapeze, the bed rail, or the head of the bed or by pushing with his feet.
      4. When using the draw sheet with an assistant, roll the draw sheet tightly under the patient on each side.
      5. Use an underhand grasp; that is, with the palms facing upwards, grasp the draw sheet at the patient's shoulder buttocks level.
      6. One assistant counts, "one, two, move." On "move," both assistants drag the draw sheet upward in bed. Do not attempt to lift the draw sheet. This is not a lifting maneuver.
      7. Your protective body mechanics involve deeping feet wide apart, pointing lead foot toward the head of the bed, keeping knees bent, pelvic tilt, holding back straight, and rocking forward onto the lead foot when dragging the draw sheet.
   D. Moving the patient in bed unassisted and without a draw sheet
      1. Ask the patient to help, if at all possible, by using the trapeze, bed rails, or head of the bed or by pushing with his feet (Fig. 5-9).
      2. Do not attempt to lift the patient. This is a dragging maneuver.
      3. Spread your legs wide and turn the lead foot toward the head of the bed.
      4. Slide one hand under the patient's shoulders and neck and grasp the opposite shoulder.
      5. Slide the other hand under the patient's waist or buttocks.

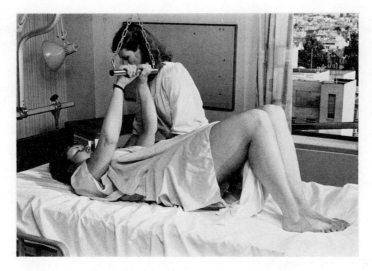

Fig. 5-9. Patient using the trapeze to move herself up in bed.

6. On a count of "one, two, move," drag the patient upward in bed by rocking over your lead foot. Secure as much of the patient's assistance as possible at this time.
7. Your protective body mechanics involve keeping knees bent, using pelvic tilt as strongly as possible, maintaining a straight back at all times, and rocking forward over your lead foot.
  E. Sitting patients on the side of the bed
1. Secure as much of the patient's assistance as possible and instruct him carefully in what you require of him.
2. Elevate the head of the bed to maximum height, if possible.
3. Turn the patient on his side facing you and drop his legs and knees over the side of the bed.
4. Slide one hand under the shoulder girdle and elevate the patient to a full sitting position.
5. Your protective body mechanics involve keeping a wide base of support, keeping knees bent, using pelvic tilt, and holding your back as straight as possible.
II. Pushing and pulling
  A. Basic body mechanics
1. Push rather than pull in all possible situations.
2. Use the pelvic tilt strongly in all of these maneuvers.
3. Maintain a wide base of support when pushing or pulling.
4. Maintain bent elbows whenever pushing, to absorb the shock that is normally translated to your spine.
  B. Pushing and pulling wheelchairs and gurneys when there is an IV stand and infusion pump inolved
1. The rules of protective body mechanics involve pelvic tilt, wide base of support, and bent elbows.
2. If you choose to push a wheelchair and infusion pump without an assistant, the patient must hold the IV stand. Both of your hands belong on the wheelchair.
3. If you must push the wheelchair with one hand and the IV stand with the other hand, the only rule of protective body mechanics left is the pelvic tilt.

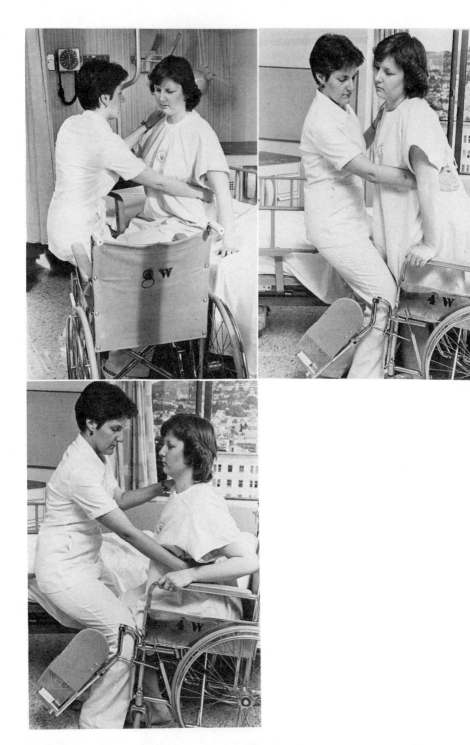

Fig. 5-10. Procedure for moving the patient from the bedside to a wheelchair with one assistant.

III. Wheelchair transfers

A. Basic body mechanics

1. The bed must be lowered to the bottom position and, if possible, the head of the bed elevated to assist the patient in sitting up.

2. The wheelchair should be placed so that it is next to the patient's strongest leg when he is sitting on the side of the bed.

3. Work only with one of the patient's legs, usually the stronger leg, to brace it during transfer activities.

4. The key to getting a patient from the bedside to a standing position is moving the head in front of the knees and keeping it there during the whole transfer activity.

B. Moving from bedside to wheelchair with one assistant (Fig. 5-10)

1. The basic body mechanics rules remain the same.

2. Get the patient sitting up on the side of the bed so that the strong leg is toward the wheelcair.

3. Stand just off center from the patient by the strongest leg.

4. Block the patient's foot with your foot and place one or both of your knees comfortably against the patient's knee.

5. Place one of your hands under the patient's axilla and around the other scapula. Place the other hand around the patient's waist. If the patient is to hold onto you at all, he holds onto your waist, not your shoulders.

6. On signal, move the patient to a standing position by rocking backward onto your rear foot and pulling the patient toward you while extending his knees. This is a tricky maneuver and requires excellent protective body mechanics. Make sure that you use the pelvic tilt strongly as you begin to move the patient and keep your knees slightly bent throughout the whole maneuver. This is a weight shifting maneuver (not back lifting) toward your body and over your rear foot.

7. When you have the patient standing and leaning against your body, pivot toward the wheelchair. This pivoting motion should occur on your rear foot. As you lower the patient into the wheelchair, do so by bending your knees and moving with the patient. Do not bend at your waist.

8. Moving from wheelchair to bed with one assistant is the same maneuver in reverse. Make sure that the wheelchair is positioned so that, as the patient stands, the strong leg is next to the bed.

C. Transfer from bed to wheelchair with two assistants

1. This transfer is for weak and debilitated patients who cannot bring themselves to a sitting or standing position. It requires a wheelchair with removable legs and sides.

2. Elevate the head of the bed as much as possible and maneuver the wheelchair in place so that it is directly opposite the patient's hips. Remove the foot pedals, knee flaps, and the closest side of the wheelchair.

3. One assistant stands at the patient's head behind the wheelchair. Hold the patient under the axilla, bringing your hands around the front and grasp his forearms. The other assistant supports the patient's lower body by holding his legs just beneath the knees.

4. On signal each assistant pulls the patient toward him and then toward the chair. The secret in this type of lift is to stretch the patient between the two assistants so that the buttocks come off the bed.

5. The protective body mechanics for the hospital personnel involve a wide base of support, a very strong pelvic tilt at the moment of accepting the patient's weight, and maximum use of the knee muscles. The assistant near the patient's head needs to employ the pelvic tilt very strongly, since there is very little opportunity for use of the knees. The assistant closer to patient's feet uses the pelvic tilt with equal strength, but has to make maximum use of his bent knees to avoid bending the trunk forward.

6. Returning the patient to bed from the wheelchair is the same type of activity.
7. When the two assistants choose not to move the patient in this manner, but to use the single assistant manner of moving him the second assistant stands to the side and assists in the standing motion.

IV. Gurney transfers
  A. Basic body mechanics
    1. The gurney should be locked in place.
    2. The bed should be equal to or a little higher than the gurney for transferring the patient from bed to gurney. The bed should be a little bit lower than the gurney for transferring the patient from gurney to bed. The assistant should use a draw sheet or mattress sheet for transferring the patient to the gurney. The patient should help, if at all possible.
    3. Body mechanics for hospital personnel involve unlocked knees at all times during the transfer. The assistant on the gurney end of the transfer should use a rocking motion onto the rear foot instead of a lifting-pulling motion with the spine. The pelvic tilt should be employed strongly by all of the transferring crew.
  B. Transfer technique with two people and a draw sheet
    1. Adjust the bed to the level of the gurney.
    2. Move the patient to the edge of the bed.
    3. Clear the draw sheet from the mattress and roll it tightly underneath the patient with the roll on the top side.
    4. Position the gurney and lock it in place.
    5. One assistant should be on the far side of the bed and his job is to keep the draw sheet taut and to clear it from the bed slightly. The other assistant should be on the gurney side and his job is to drag the draw sheet over to the gurney using a rocking motion over the rear foot.
    6. One of the assistants should be the captain and count "one, two, move." On "move," the assistant on the bed side pulls the draw sheet tight and lifts slightly while the assistant on the gurney side pulls with a rocking motion. Move the patient to the gurney in sections. Do not attempt to move the patient all the way out to the gurney with the first pull.
    7. When one assistant finds himself bending over the bed or the gurney in a lifting or pulling manner, the pelvic tilt is the only method of protective body mechanics that keeps the spine safe.
  C. Transfer from bed to stretcher with an able patient using the trapeze
    1. The rules for protective body mechanics remain the same.
    2. Two assistants are involved, but stand at the head and the foot end of the gurney.
    3. The patient takes hold of the trapeze and elevates his upper body from the bed.
    4. The assistant at the foot end of the gurney takes hold of the legs and move them onto the gurney first.
    5. The assistant at the head end of the gurney then moves the head and upper trunk onto the gurney.
    6. Protective body mechanics employed during this maneuver involve the pelvic tilt, a wide base of support, and a rocking motion from one foot to the other while carrying the weight.
    7. Returning to bed uses the same procedure.
  D. Moving from bed to gurney or gurney to bed with four assistants
    1. The body mechanics for this maneuver remain the same.
    2. Two of the assistants are on the gurney side when the patient is being moved to the gurney. One assistant is at the head of the bed and the other assistant is at the side of the bed opposite to where the gurney is situated.
    3. The draw sheet is employed in the same manner as before.

4. The assistants on the gurney side pull the draw sheet to them using the pelvic tilt, knee bend, and rocking concept of body mechanics, while the assistant at the far end of the bed simply keeps the draw sheet taut and follows the patient as the maneuver is accomplished. The assistant at the head of the bed clears the head and the shoulder from the bed and ensures that the head and shoulder move carefully onto the gurney.

5. Moving from gurney to bed is the same maneuver.

E. Using the patient roller for transferring from bed to gurney

1. This requires two assistants. Move the patient to the edge of the bed and push the stretcher in place.

2. Place the Davis roller half on the bed and half on the gurney lengthwise. Cover it with a long sheet.

3. Place the patient and the draw sheet on one edge of the Davis roller and proceed along the same lines as a two-person bed-to-gurney transfer.

4. The body mechanics involve a wide base of support, bent knees, and pelvic tilt throughout the maneuver.

5. The pulling movement is a rocking motion over the rear foot rather than a lifting action with the back.

6. Leave the pillow in place if the patient has long hair. If the pillow is not left in place, be sure that the hair does not become trapped between the sheets or in the roller mechanism.

F. Using the Surgie Lift

1. The instructions for using the Surgie Lift are the same as for using any other rolling device. Keep the knees slightly bent, use the pelvic tilt, and avoid overextending yourself during pushing or pulling activities.

2. While pulling the Surgie Lift canvas under the patient, maintain a pelvic tilt.

G. Pushing gurneys and other wheeled stretchers

1. When one person pushes the gurney or stretcher, the pelvic tilt is the most important of the body mechanics for protecting the spine.

2. A wide base of support is necessary for adequate pushing power.

3. The arm should remain slightly bent to absorb some of the shock.

4. When turning corners, stay close to the gurney and use a wide base of support, keep your knees slightly bent, and maintain a strong pelvic tilt.

5. When two people are pushing a gurney, the rules remain the same.

V. Patient lifting problems

A. Basic body mechanics

1. The most important rule for hospital personnel to remember in problem lifting situations is to stay safe themselves.

2. The object of any problem lifting sequence is to get the patient in a position of mechanical advantage for you. Get as much as is needed to lift the patient.

3. The pelvic tilt is the only rule of body mechanics that keeps you safe during the whole lift.

B. The disabled patient on the floor, open access

1. This is one of the easier lifts to perform in the problem lifting routine.

2. There are many ways to lift the patient. If three or more assistants are present, a doubled long sheet may be used as a stretcher. Pull the sheet under the patient or roll him onto the sheet and roll it as tight as possible. Two assistants are at the shoulder section of the patient, one on either side, and one assistant should be at the foot section. All assistants are in a squatting position with an underhand grip on the sheet. One of the assistants is the captain and counts, "one, two, lift." On "lift," all three lift the patient up and move him to the bed. Maintaining a wide base of support, a pelvic tilt, and a spine as straight as possible are the body mechanics to use in protecting yourself during this lift.

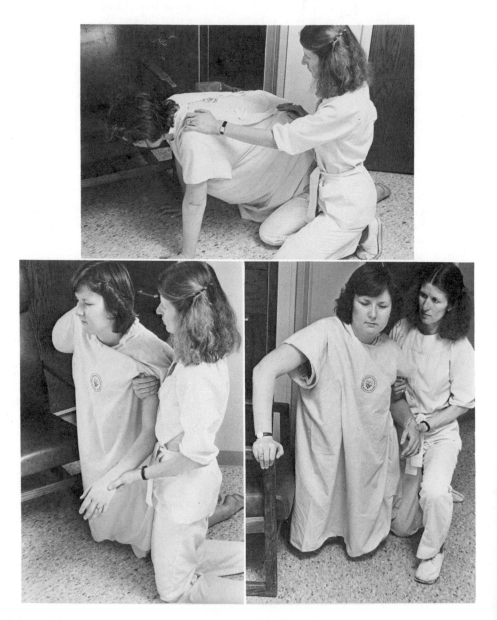

Fig. 5-11. Procedure for lifting the bad back patient from the floor in an open area.

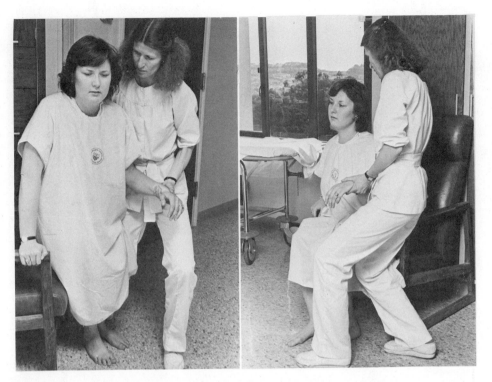

Fig. 5-11, cont'd. Procedure for lifting the bad back patient from the floor in an open area.

3. When only two assistants are available, a lift out of a wheelchair may be attempted. One of the assistants moves to the patient's head and sits him up, assuming an underhand grip beneath the patient's axilla and in front on the forearms. The assistant nearer the legs flexes the knees and gets a good grasp under them. On the count of "one, two, lift," both assistants lift the patient, drawing him taut between them and moving toward the chair or the bed. The rules of protective body mechanics involve the use of a pelvic tilt throughout the entire activity, maintaining a wide base of support, and keeping the back as vertical or upright as possible.

4. When only one person is available, the lift becomes much more difficult (Fig. 5-11). If the patient is conscious and able to assist, it is best to try to get him up in stages. Pull a chair close to the patient's strong side. Turn him over on his stomach. Attempt to get him in an "all-fours" crawling position using a firm grip about his waist. When the patient is in an all-fours position, draw the chair close to him and have him put at least one of his arms on the chair. It is now easy for you to assist the patient to a half-standing position with a grip around his waist. Half turn the patient from this position and seat him in the chair. Once he is sitting in the chair, it is then easy to get him into the bed. The protective body mechanics to remember during this whole procedure involve using a wide base of support, a very strong pelvic tilt, and maintaining the back as vertical and straight as possible.

C. The disabled patient on the floor in a confined space (e.g., a bathroom)

1. The basic body mechanics remain the same during this whole procedure, that is, a wide base of support, a strong pelvic tilt, bent knees, and vertical or straight back.

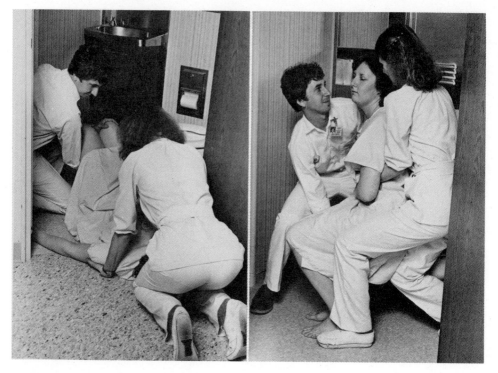

Fig. 5-12. Procedure for lifting the bad back patient from the floor in the bathroom using the chair lift.

2. This is a rather difficult lift for one person to attempt. It is probably best to drag the patient out of the bathroom and then try to help.
3. When two assistants are available, both may get close to the patient and use the chair lift, one assistant at the patient's head and one at his knees. Lift the patient onto the commode, into the wheelchair, or carry him out of the bathroom (Fig. 5-12).
4. A draw sheet may be used, if the patient is unconscious and unable to respond.
5. The motions to avoid in confined lifting spaces are bending over without bending the knees, moving faster than is normal in this type of situation, and acting with jerky or quick motions that are not in unison with the lifting team.

6 BACK SCHOOL IN THE HOME ENVIRONMENT

There are many specific changes that a person can make in the home environment to protect and thus allow his back to heal after an injury. The basic principles are to keep the back at rest most of the time, to avoid extreme positions of the spine for accomplishing activities, and to keep the forces on the spine to a minimum.

BED REST
Proper lying position

The proper state for the spine during bed rest is a contour position, either lying on the back with pillows under the knees, or lying on the side with the knees curled up in a fetal position (Fig. 6-1). This same position can be accomplished on a couch. When lying on the side, it is a good idea to keep a pillow under the waist, so that the spine does not sag into the surface on which you are lying.

Lying on the abdomen can cause excessive lumbar lordosis and be painful or damaging. It is best, if one has to lie in this position, to have a pillow under the abdomen to take the sway out of the back.

Bedding

Soft mattresses can cause the spine to sag and produce considerable strain on a vertebral segment. This is the reason for a firm mattress. Lying flat on the back on a firm surface, however, can arch or extend the lumbar spine excessively. The weight of the legs tips the pelvis anteriorly on the spine.

Waterbeds are questionable as to their value for low back pain patients. Some patients do well with them and others do not. It probably is related to the position in which a patient sleeps and the way his weight is distributed. If a patient has heavy buttocks that sag deeply into a waterbed, causing excessive swayback, the painful back might get worse. If the waterbed has too little water, it can also cause more sagging. A side-sleeper or belly-sleeper is liable to have more sagging in the waterbed than a back sleeper. There have not been any good, well-controlled studies that verify the value of a waterbed. It is simply a matter of personal experience. We advise patients to try waterbed, either in a motel or rental situation, to be sure that their condition improves, or at least does not get worse, before purchasing one.

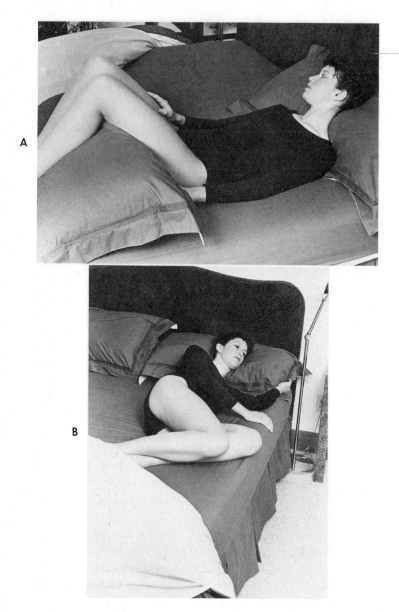

Fig. 6-1. Proper position for spine during bed rest is, **A,** lying on the back with pillows under knees or, **B,** fetal position.

Acute low back pain

Bed rest can be therapeutic and there is a way that it should be used with each patient's condition. During the acute phases of low back pain, such as an anulus tear or nerve root inflammation, lying down lowers the intradiscal pressure and places the spine in a position of safety. This is usually a contour position, although with some disc problems the position of extension is indicated. In the comfortable, safe, and nontraumatic position, the underlying inflammatory process has a chance to heal. It may take hours for this to occur. The patient should remain in bed until he can safely, with his own knowledge, strength, and body mechanics, move on to other activities. A very knowledgeable and strong individual can move out of bed quickly with a minor anulus or facet problem. Severely contused or swollen nerve roots can take days to heal, even with the addition of cortisone.

Chronic low back pain

More chronic degenerative lumbar segment problems require periods of rest each day in a safe and nontraumatic position to allow the low-grade inflammation to resolve. Normal daily activities on a degenerating or unstable spinal segment lead to low-grade inflammation. If the individual does not rest, the inflammation continues to build until it reaches proportions that are painful. With periods of rest, either at night or at various times during the day, the segment has a chance to repair itself and the inflammation has an opportunity to subside before it reaches a painful level.

Exercising during bed rest

There are, of course, problems with long periods of bed rest. There are physiological changes that occur with nonweight bearing and lack of normal use of the body. Exercises can be done at bed rest to maintain strength, so that when the resting period is over, muscle tone and coordination are adequate for getting out of bed. At any time, while in bed in a contour position, the abdominal muscles can be tightened and buttocks squeezed together. This is essentially a pelvic tilt exercise (Chapter 4). By isometrically holding this position, the patient is strengthening his muscles. Habit patterns can be developed in this fashion, so that when the patient begins to move out of bed, he can move the same muscular contractions to help immobilize the spine, while the arms and legs do the positioning for the trunk.

Other exercises can also be done in bed, while maintaining a pelvic tilt position. The patient can use small weights or springs in bed. He can use an overhead trapeze or various other resistive exercise aids to develop strength in all of the extremities. Another exercise that can assist in maintaining back health care is straight leg raising. The patient pulls his knee to his chest by placing his hands behind his thigh. He then straightens his knee, thus stretching the hamstrings and sciatic nerve (Fig. 6-2). This of course, should not be done if very painful. Keeping the hamstrings lengthened makes proper bending and lifting easier. There are other specialized exercises that can be done at bed rest, such as press-ups or lumbar extension exercises. These are used specifically for acute disc problems, and are thought to relieve posterior anulus edema and nucleus migration (Fig. 6-3).

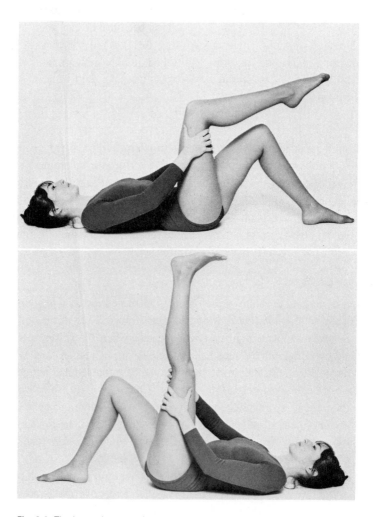

Fig. 6-2. The hamstring stretch.

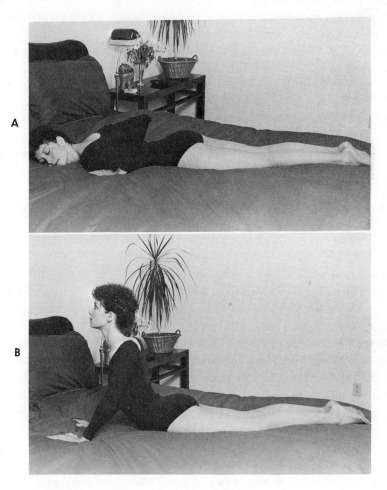

Fig. 6-3. McKenzie "press-up." **A,** Step one. **B,** Step two.

Getting out of bed

Getting out of bed can be damaging and painful to the spine. Unless a person has strong abdominal muscles and is generally in good physical shape, he should not simple come to a sitting position from lying supine. Doing so generally causes the spine to go into full flexion under considerable force. Using the hands to pull up on an overhead bar or pushup from the side is safer, but awkward. It is much easier to roll onto the side, tighten the abdomen, and push to to a sitting position, as the legs are slipped over the edge of the bed or couch (Fig. 6-4). The abdomen should be held tight during all of these types of maneuvers. It is good to do some exercises in bed before getting up, to assure strength and coordination in these maneuvers. A few pelvic tilts and abdominal setting exercises can be done quite well in bed.

SITTING

Once the patient advances past the bed rest phase, sitting is one of the most common activities. The patient pushes himself up from a lying position and is now sitting on the side of the bed. Because the spine is still sensitive to bearing full sitting weight with its high intradiscal pressures and frequent aggravation of back pain conditions, sitting at this time requires additional support. The most available support at this position is having the arms and elbows extended, supporting some of the weight of the body on the hands. Leaning back against something gives additional spinal support (Fig. 6-5).

Proper sitting position

Sitting is less stressful on the spine, if the back of the seat against which the patient reclines is at approximately 120 degrees to the surface on which his buttocks and thighs rest. Generally the lumbar spine should not be allowed to sag into full flexion in a soft cushion or pillow. A firm back with some additional lumbar support is usually most comfortable. It is also best if the knees are elevated from the hip joints (Fig. 6-5). The exact position of comfort and least stress is different with each pathological condition and physical makeup. The physician or therapist can help the patient identify this position, and the patient can quickly determine which position is most agreeable to him. It sometimes takes several hours in a particular position before the patient can determine that it produces some discomfort. Some positions immediately cause pain and therefore should be avoided. While the patient is at bed rest, the bed can be adjusted to various contour and sitting positions with pillows and whatever facility is available. Back supports can be fashioned. The patient can remain in these contour sitting positions for hours at a time to test his comfort. The same positions can then be simulated, once the patient is out of bed, by using couches, contour chairs, chaise lounges, etc.

Getting in and out of a seated position

Getting in and out of a seated position requires that the spine be immobilized by the surrounding musculature. This entails tightening the abdomen, doing a pelvic tilt, and using the arms and legs to position the trunk so that lumbar motion is not necessary (Fig. 6-6). Use the hip joints rather than the lumbar segments to accomplish any bending of the

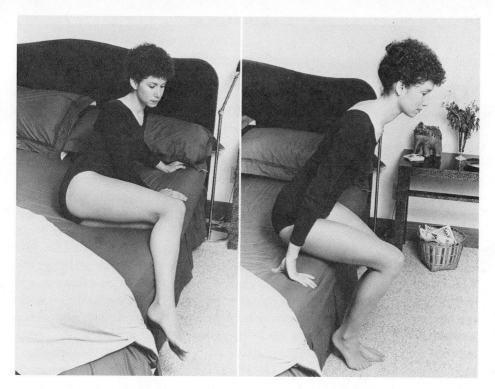

Fig. 6-4. Getting out of bed correctly.

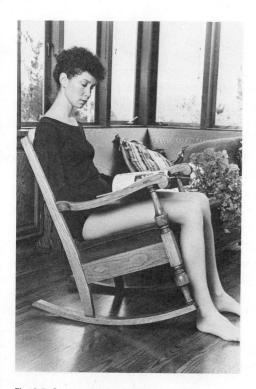

Fig. 6-5. Correct sitting position.

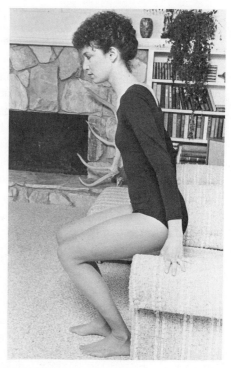

Fig. 6-6. Getting out of a chair.

trunk on the thighs. This again brings us to one of the major principles in all of body mechanics.

The normal way of bending for the human spine is to use the lumbar segments first and the hip joints second. It is not a natural phenomenon for most individuals in an industrialized society to hold the lumbar segments rigid, while freeing the hip joints, for all bending activities. Such a method of body mechanics essentially amounts to lengthening the lever arm of the trunk, as it plays against the lever arm of the lower extremities. This requires considerably more muscular force and energy to accomplish tasks. It also greatly increases the force across the hip joints. If there are already painful problems with the hips, such body mechanics maneuvers may not be possible. It is not known what effects such body mechanics will have on the hip joints over long periods of time. By the time most of us are required to learn this type of body mechanics, our spines are so painful and degenerated that we must be willing to trade some potential long-range effects of the hip joints for immediate relief of a painful spine. If the patient learns to balance the use of the lumbar spine against the use of the hip joints, so that neither are overused, perhaps we could greatly reduce both hip and low back disease. It is my feeling, although far from scientifically validated, that there is a basic overuse of the spine in patients who develop early and severe low back pain. This may have to do with early training and learning. It may also have to do with some inflexibility of the hip joints or tightness of the hamstrings, which encourages overuse of the lumbar spine. If such errors in body mechanics could be identified early in life, perhaps they could be corrected and the incidence of low back pain greatly reduced.

Sitting in straight back chairs

Sitting in straight back chairs does not give adequate low back support. With considerable muscular effort a person can hold himself erect and prevent sagging into lumbar flexion, which so greatly increases the intradiscal pressure. Such muscular efforts, however, rarely continue for very long. The patient begins to relax and slump or sag forward into lumbar flexion. Most low back disc problems are aggravated by such a position. The patient then attempts to stand and passes from full lumbar flexion into nearly full extension. The sitting position makes temporary changes in the disc and facet joints in such a way that passing into a full range of extension creates pain. There are many theoretical reasons for such pain. There may be a posterior migration of nuclear material in the disc, edema may be developing in the posterior aspects of the disc and anulus tears, and facet joints are being stretched and possibly malaligned. Whatever the cause, this change in position from sitting in flexion to standing is one of the most common complaints of low back pain patients. It can be totally prevented by not sitting in a full flexion position, by using low back support, by maintaining the contour position and by substituting hip flexion for lumbar flexion.

Sitting on the ground

Sitting on the ground has been advocated by many specialists in the field of low back pain. (Fig. 6-7). The ground-dwelling population seems to have less low back pain than

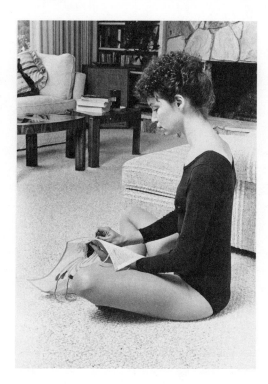

Fig. 6-7. Sitting on the ground.

that in industrialized countries. This has led to research in the effects of sitting on the ground. Beneficial effects may be as simple as sharing the load between the front and the back of the disc. Perhaps sitting on the ground in full lumbar flexion keeps the pressure on the anterior aspects of the disc for much of the time. This is in contradistinction to the industrialized countries, where the erect posture leads to long-range pressures on the posterior aspects of the discs. It is these posterior aspects that seem to deteriorate first. This is most likely caused by mechanical pressures and poor nutrition and circulation. Anulus tears and disc ruptures occur with mechanical pressures and the higher stresses developed in the posterior aspects of the discs with bending, lifting, and twisting activities. Whatever the reason, there seems to be some long-range protective value in sitting on the ground. This seems to be most valuable when done before the degenerative segment develops. Many feel that sitting on the ground can be accomplished and is of great value, even after degenerative segment disease develops. If it is practiced after low back pain develops, it should be done carefully, slowly, and painlessly.

Sitting in motor vehicles

It is well known that sitting in automobiles, trucks, or anything that vibrates leads to back pain. Long periods of sitting should be broken up with periods of walking, using the

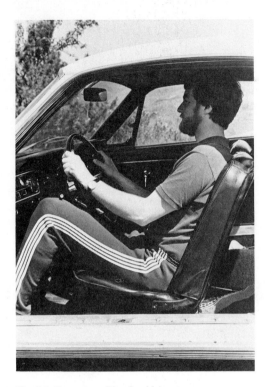

Fig. 6-8. Contour position for driving a car.

full range of motion of the lumbar spine, particularly in extension. Such breaks in constant positioning apparently allow recovery of elasticity, hydration, nutrition, circulation, and normal anatomy. The driver should sit in a contour position (Fig. 6-8).

Sitting for long periods

The patient returning to a job that requires mostly sitting should practice long periods of sitting at home. He should be thoroughly educated in the back school with regard to the types of chairs that are available, especially the Ergon chair, the Vertebra chair, the Ricarro seat, and the Barca lounger. He should have the opportunity to see some of these special types of chairs and to sit in them for periods of time. He might even want to purchase one for his own use when he returns to work. He should be educated in the ways to adjust these chairs so that his spine is most comfortable and in an acceptable position for his medical condition. When used properly a chair can provide mobility, support, and comfort in many positions. Chairs at home can be adjusted to simulate a good office chair. With a firm pillow behind the lumbosacral spine, the patient can sit and work at home for several hours simulating his working conditions. If he is not comfortable, further training must be accomplished before he returns to his usual occupation. When he does return to his usual work, it should be for a few hours at first, if possible, to see what problems have been overlooked in his working area. He should determine whether he is having any pain. He can then work for half a day and eventually a full day. Even if he goes to work and simply takes care of some of his personal business without having an official return to work notice, it is far better than going to work for the first time for 8 hours and being vulnerable to circumstances that may cause a recurrence of his condition.

There are many supports that can be purchased to convert a conventional chair to one that is more acceptable by body mechanics standards. Some of these are inflatable and others are made of metal that is bendable and moldable to the position that is most comfortable and appropriate for the patient's spinal pathology. These types of supports can be folded up and carried by the patient. Some even have handles and look like briefcases. They can be taken on airplanes, on buses, and to meetings in which a patient might have to sit for hours in an otherwise catastrophic position. In the back school a patient can be placed in a room with various cushions, triangles of styrofoam and foam rubber, beanbags and other types of cushions and he is told to find a position that is most comfortable. The position that he seeks is helpful in his diagnosis, as well as developing apropriate furniture for him at home and at work. This is a form of surveillance and is helpful in confirming his diagnosis. If there is no position that is comfortable under any circumstances, we may be dealing with some neoplastic or infectious disease that is not related to position or activity. The other possibility is that the patient has some secondary gain or psychological problem, which leaves him unwilling to be comfortable under any circumstance.

STANDING AND WALKING

Standing in a static position is potentially as detrimental as sitting in full flexion. Standing erect creates a position of extension of the lumbar spine, which transfers the forces of the vertebral segment to the posterior aspects of the disc and to the facet joints. If there is pathology and pain emanating from these posterior structures, the position can be painful. By doing a pelvic tilt, the lumbosacral angle and lumbar lordosis are reduced. Therefore, the forces on the posterior disc and facet joints are reduced. It is difficult and awkward to maintain a pelvic tilt position with both feet together in an erect posture. It is more natural to flex one hip by placing a foot on a stool or other elevation of approximately 6 to 10 inches. This creates a pelvic tilt that does not require constant muscular efforts to maintain. Since walking is a series of flexing the hip, pelvic tilt is being used most of the time. This reduces the strain on the posterior aspect of the vertebral segment.

Periods of standing can be broken up with stretching exercises with full lumbar flexion and extension. This must be done carefully and painlessly (Fig. 6-9). While standing in an erect position, the patient can lean forward and support himself on a counter with his elbows or outstretched arms. This provides lumbar flexion as well as a form of traction that further reduces intradiscal pressure and the forces on the painful lumbar segment.

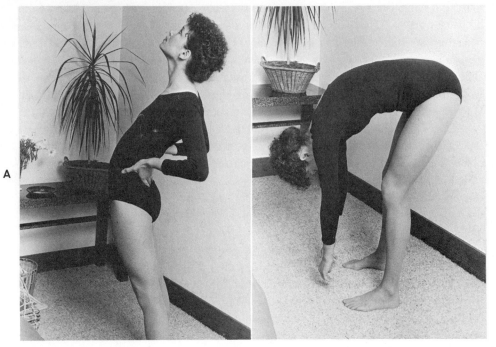

A   B

Fig. 6-9. Stretching exercises. **A,** "Extension" exercise. **B,** Advanced stretch.

DAILY ACTIVITIES
Home self-care

We can now apply the principles of lying down, sitting, standing, and walking, as well as the previous chapter on principles of body mechanics, to a patient's daily activities. The low back pain patient rests at night in a comfortable atraumatic position. He gets out of bed properly after a few exercises and allows a period of time for his spinal segments to adjust before getting into any significant bending activities. The patient does not stand in a single position, but walks about, perhaps takes a hot shower, and gradually loosens up his spine with progressive flexion and extension exercises.

A moderate walk is a good exercise and tests the patient's current spinal status. If the spine does not seem ready for normal daily activities, a corset could be used. If pain is present, alteration of the daily plan may have to be made to include more prolonged exercise, mobilization, traction, or bracing.

The positions that are known to recreate the patient's pain are avoided. When bending forward at the sink to brush his teeth or wash his face, the patient does not use lumbar flexion, but uses hip flexion and supports himself on his hand or elbow (Fig. 6-10). When sitting on the toilet, the patient should not allow himself to slump into a full lumbar-flexion position, but should support himself with his hands or with his musculature in a fairly erect position or should flex forward from the hips with his elbows on his knees (Fig. 6-11).

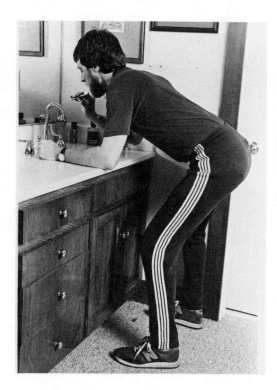

Fig. 6-10. Posture for bending forward at the sink.

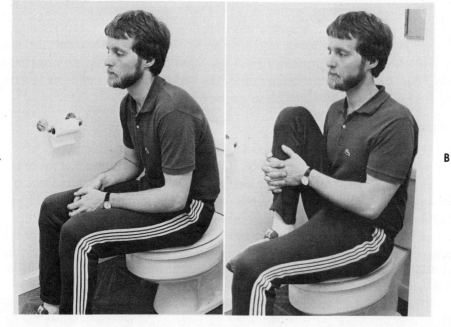

Fig. 6-11. Sitting on the toilet. **A**, Wrong. **B**, One method of support.

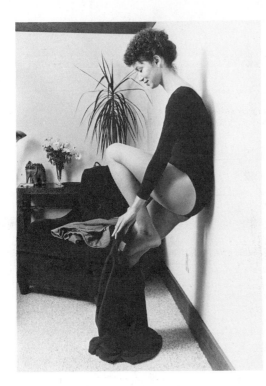

Fig. 6-12. Position for dressing.

In getting dressed, the patient should not bend over to put on his shoes, socks, or trousers. He should lean back against the wall or lie down, keeping his back flat as he uses his hips and knees to position his feet for the appropriate dressing maneuvers (Fig. 6-12). A few stretching or strengthening exercises before getting dressed or taking on any significant working activities assure him that he has good control of his spine and knows the level of capabilities he is likely to accomplish.

Household activities

The back pain patient rests in bed until he is free from pain. He then gets out of bed, and with the use of excellent body mechanics, attends to his personal hygiene and feeds himself. If he is unable to do this painlessly, he should remain at bed rest and seek further medical attention. Either he is doing these activities improperly, he is not strong enough or knowledgeable enough in the body mechanics for these activities, or his condition is so severe that these activities cannot be done. If the latter is the case, the patient should probably be in the hospital having further diagnostic tests and more aggressive medical evaluation and treatment. Assuming, however, that he is able to accomplish his home self-care painlessly, he is ready for increased activity.

The patient should be able to safely and painlessly get into a automobile and adjust his seat to a comfortable position, using the information previously given for sitting instructions. To accomplish other activities he can drive or be driven for distances that

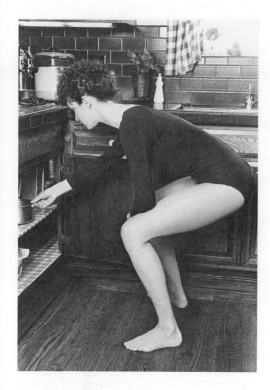

Fig. 6-13. Position for bending over to get to a low cupboard.

take up to 30 minutes. He should go to a back school and receive further information and training with regard to advancing his activities, strength, and body mechanics.

Household chores should be done with a good understanding of what positions aggravate and relieve pain. Spinal movements should be maintained within the pain-free range by proper body mechanics. Bending forward to pick up things should be accomplished with the knees and hips and not the spine (Fig. 6-13). Reaching should be done not by extending the spine to full lordosis, but by maintaining pelvic tilt and stepping up on a stool. Vacuuming should be done by a forward and backward motion with the hips and knees rather than the lumbar spine. Furniture should not be moved that cannot be handled comfortably with a straight backbend, using the hip and knees. Work that requires standing in one place, such as ironing, should be organized so that the back can be placed at rest against a wall or at least by having one foot up on a stool or a book (Fig. 6-14, *A* and *B*). Work at ground level should be done by either sitting or kneeling on the ground with the spine in a fairly neutral position, avoiding full flexion.

The patient can accomplish kitchen activities by standing at a sink with his foot up on a low stool or telephone book (Fig. 6-15). He can lean against the refrigerator or wall while he is waiting for his coffee or talking on the phone (Fig. 6-16). He can then sit in a kitchen chair with good back support or lean forward on the table with his arm or elbow (Fig. 6-17). He does not sit for more than a few minutes before getting up and taking a short walk.

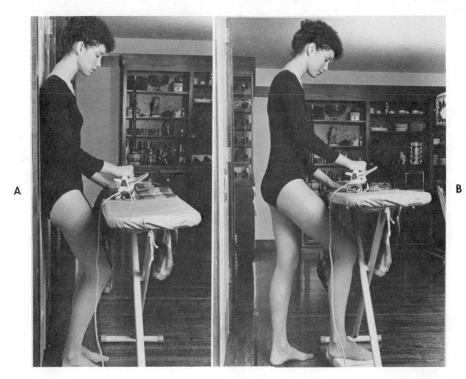

Fig. 6-14. Two ways of ironing. **A,** Back resting against wall. **B,** One foot up resting on an object.

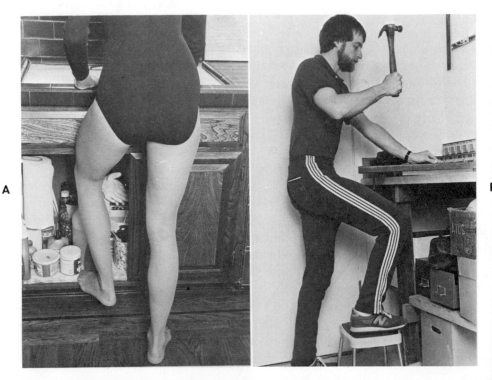

Fig. 6-15. Position for standing while working at, **A,** kitchen counter and, **B,** workbench.

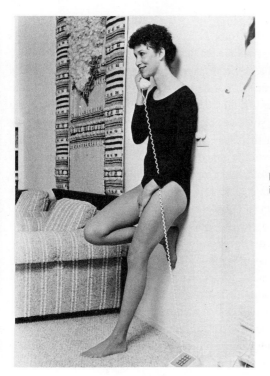

Fig. 6-16. Resting position when standing and talking on the telephone.

Fig. 6-17. Sitting position in a kitchen chair.

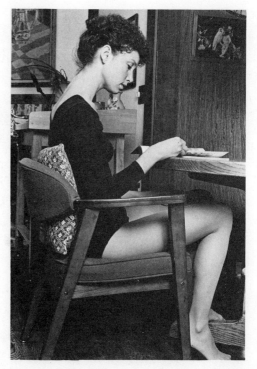

Lifting

Because the patient needs to go to the store, he should be instructed with regard to lifting, carrying, and particularly placing packages in the trunk of the car. Bending for this activity is quite tricky. A person is unable to bend from the knees because he would then be pushed away from the trunk of the car and not have access to it. Therefore, he has to bend over from the hips, with his knees straight. He can rest his hand or elbow on the trunk of the car for additional support. Some people are even able to put one foot in the trunk of the car or on the bumper and then lean against their knee for protection and support (Fig. 6-18). This is the principle of the straight backbend, which can be applied to many other situations, such as getting your luggage from a baggage claim area at a bus depot or airplane terminal. However, this bend is rather complicated and needs a fair amount of practice and instruction for most people to accomplish.

Any patient should be able to quickly learn a conventional safe type of bend and lift. He usually does this type of a bend and lift because it is the least painful during the acute phase. This conventional safe lift consists of getting directly over the object to be lifted and straddling it with his feet. Then he squats down, bending his knees and hips, keeping his back straight. He grasps the object with his arms extended and then goes straight up. Although this is a safe bend, it is somewhat awkward compared to the golfer getting his golf ball out of the cup or the athlete picking up a ball on the run (Fig. 6-19 *A* and *B*).

There are other ways of bending, which are not particularly dangerous, if a person is coordinated and strong. The advanced type of bending and lifting can be taught in the back school as the patient's strength and body mechanics improve.

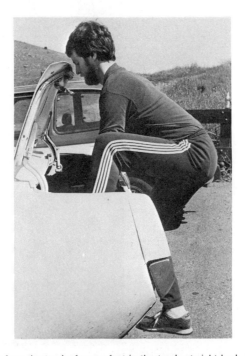

Fig. 6-18. Lifting an object from the trunk of a car: foot in the trunk, straight back, knee bent.

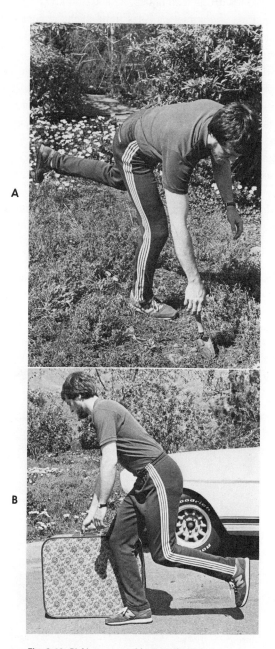

Fig. 6-19. Picking up an object on the run.

Carrying

The patient now has to carry things from his car to his home and around the house (Fig. 6-20). Similar to his lifting techniques, he needs to keep the load close to his body, his back straight, and his abdominal muscles tight. If the patient can remember the one rule of keeping his abdominal muscles tight during all changes of position, he would almost be safe from further injury. As previously stated, when he gets up from a lying down position, he tightens his abdomen and pushes himself up to a sitting position. When he goes from a sitting position to a standing position, he should tighten his abdominal muscles and stand up. He should not bend at the lumbar segment or relax his abdominal muscles until he finds a good balanced position in which the spine is safe. The more external support that he can find, the better off he is when he relieves his stomach muscles of their job. He can be leaning back against the wall or leaning forward on his elbows before he allows his stomach muscles to release. This is the value of the timed endurance abdominal partial sit-up and isometric abdominal holding exercise. If a patient is able to hold his abdominal muscles tight in a partial sit-up for 4 or 5 minutes, then he is certainly able to be on his feet and hold his abdominal muscles tight as he walks or carries something for up to 4 or 5 minutes before he puts the object down or finds a position of rest.

In carrying loads that are asymmetrical or need to be carried out to the side, extra

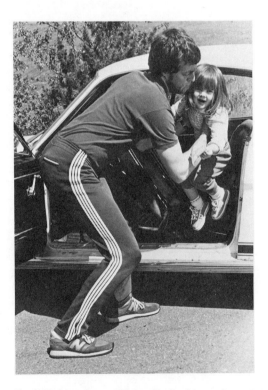

Fig. 6-20. Removing a child from the back seat of an automobile.

education is necessary. It is better to carry an object on the shoulders or even on the head, rather than in one hand, when that might force the patient into a lateral bending position while ambulating. The object can also be carried in front with two hands.

The spine should not be allowed to fall into swayback or extension while carrying a heavy load. Maintaining a pelvic tilt prevents this. Leaning forward in lumbar flexion while carrying a load can also be quite dangerous. As the hip and abdominal muscles fatigue while protecting the spine from flexion, eventually the lumbar vertebrae are in sufficient flexion to increase intradiscal pressure and threaten further posterior disc tears, posterior nucleus migration, and even herniation.

Heavier work around the house

A patient may want to try out some heavier work around the house before returning to a job, particularly one that is going to require 8 hours of relatively heavy work. He should therefore progressively increase his activities at home, finding jobs that are fairly difficult to do. Vacuuming is a fairly strenuous job that requires a good knowledge of body mechanics. The abdominal muscles must be tightened throughout the entire maneuver, with periods of rest. The knees must be bent most of the time, again requiring ability for long endurance of quadriceps. This is the reason for the timed progressive wall slide exercise. If a patient can achieve 3 or 4 minutes of wall slide, he can tolerate 3 or 4

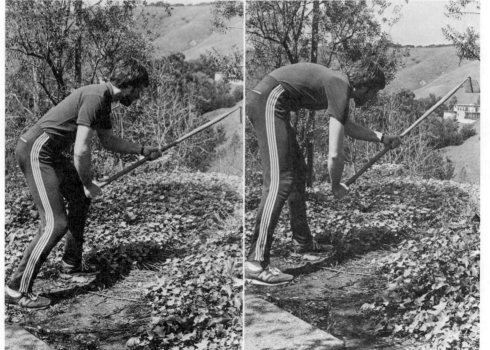

Fig. 6-21. Hoeing in the garden. **A,** Right: back straight, abdomen tight, knees bent. **B,** Wrong: back bent, knees straight.

minutes of heavy partially squatting activities, such as vacuuming. With the abdomen tight and the knees bent, the patient can force his weight forward and back, propelling the vacuum cleaner with his legs, while his spine stays immobilized and supported with the tight abdominal musculature. If there is a need to bend, the bend must come from the hips and not from the spine.

Gardening is a body mechanics activity similar to vacuuming. Using rakes, hoes, and wheelbarrows requires essentially the same body mechanics (Fig. 6-21). Bending down to the ground to do weeding and trowel work is a bit more difficult. If a patient has very stretched-out hamstrings and a good knowledge of body mechanics, he can get to the ground, as many of the field workers do, without injuring his back. He needs to bend over at the hips, keeping his back straight.

Most individuals in industralized countries, however, are not in that kind of physical shape and do not have the background and training for such activities. Therefore they need to get to the ground by other means, which involves sitting or kneeling. When sitting or kneeling, the protective functions of the knee are eliminated and you have only the hip joints to bend, rather than the spine. In kneeling, a person can flex forward at the hips and support himself with one hand, thus being in a crawling position and working with the other hand (Fig. 6-22, *A*). The spine can be kept straight and even extended in that

A

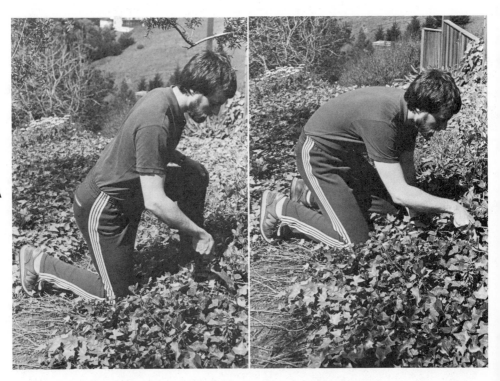

Fig. 6-22. Working in the garden, kneeling. **A,** Right: back straight. **B,** Wrong: good support with hand but too much backbend.

position. Also in the kneeling position the patient can sit back on his haunches or lean back against his heels, keeping his spine straight and using a tool with a handle on it to work on the ground in front and to the side of him (Fig. 6-22, *B*).

Sitting is worse than kneeling because it then eliminates both the knees and the hip joints, leaving only the spine to do the positioning. You have to sit fairly still without slumping forward and work to the side within an arm's reach (Fig. 6-23). The fortunate patient who does not have pain with flexion of the lumbar spine may be comfortable and even feel better stretching forward by squatting or leaning and working in a fully flexed lumbar position. Great care must be used, however, when working in this position. Loading the spine in a fully flexed position with rotation is again the most probable cause of anulus tears and herniated lumbar discs.

Pushing a lawn mower is similar to pushing a vacuum cleaner but requires more physical effort. Carpentry requires getting to the ground in a similar manner to gardening. Chopping wood requires a rather special form of body mechanics with good coordination. The abdomen must be held tight and the knees bent, while the ax is thrown with the shoulders, using as minimal rotation of the spine as possible. The force to break the wood comes from the arms and a thrust of the fixed spine and pelvis on the hips.

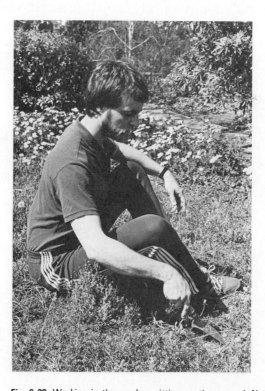

Fig. 6-23. Working in the garden, sitting on the ground. Note straight back.

Awkward positions

There are activities around the home that require difficult or awkward positions. These awkward positions, which are most often found while doing plumbing work, electrical wiring, and automobile mechanics type of activities, require contortions of the body that can put the spine in a dangerous or painful position (Fig. 6-24). There are ways to achieve these positions without using the spine. If a patient can learn to use the basic rule of immobilizing the spine first and then using the hips, knees, and shoulders to get where he needs to go to do his work, he will do fine (Fig. 6-25, *A* and *B*). For example, getting under a cabinet or small shelf to do plumbing or electrical work, the patient should lie flat on the floor or on an otherwise level surface, tighten his abdomen, and bend his knees. His spine is now safe as he tightens his abdomen before bending his shoulders and neck to get to the position where he can do his work. If he has to bend around corners, he must make the angle of the bend at the hips, rather than at the lumbar spine. This may mean crawling fully into a cabinet with the chest and abdomen at the angle of the cabinet and pressing against the groin and hip joints. Working under an automobile is similarly done flat on the back with the knees bent, if possible. The abdominal muscles are tightened and the patient reaches up to do the work with his arms and shoulders. In leaning over the fender of a car, the patient should bend over from the hips (Fig. 6-26). If his legs are not long enough, he should stand on a stool or box so that he can lean and rest his abdomen over the fender with his back fully straight and his abdominal muscles tightened during the whole procedure. This may take a longer period of time because of the patient's endurance but these new habits are what is going to prevent further progression of his disease and the pain, which he has not been understanding.

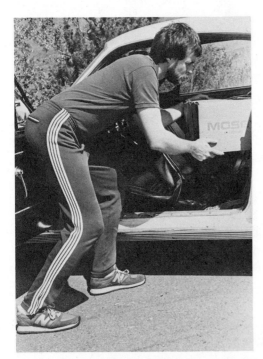

Fig. 6-24. Awkward position for removing an object from a car.

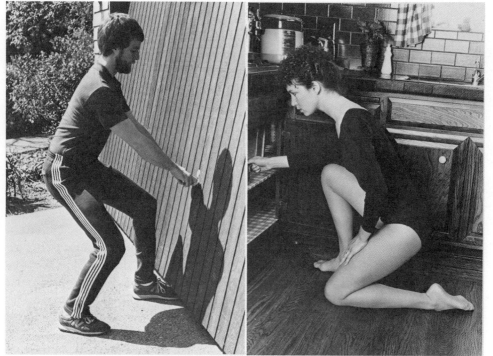

Fig. 6-25. Correct body mechanics for, **A,** opening garage door and, **B,** getting into lower cabinet.

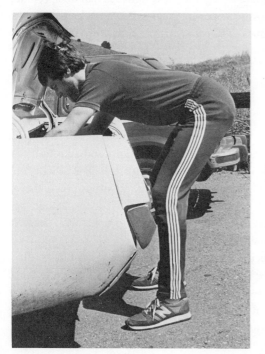

Fig. 6-26. Correct body mechanics for leaning over the fender of a car.

Climbing and reaching

We all have a tendency to be lazy when reaching. We stand on our tiptoes and reach as high as we can. This throws our lumbar spine into a swayback or extension that can be painful and detrimental with certain lumbar spinal conditions, especially those of facet disease and spondylolysis. The body mechanics for this activity are as simple as getting close to the work to be done by obtaining a lift such as a chair, stool, or ladder. The stability of such a lift is fairly important. For a patient with a precarious back, a fall or sudden jolt could do considerable damage and start the patient's symptoms anew. The size of the lift is also important. Stepping up on a small lift is similar to climbing stairs. It takes little lumbar flexion to climb up. The patient can simply tighten his abdominal muscles and do a pelvic tilt, while placing one leg on the lift and then pushing vertically up to that level. Going down can cause extension of the lumbar spine and some trauma. With good quadriceps muscles one leg can be placed forward, while the leg that remains on the lift or stair flexes, maintaining the balance and lowering the body with the use of the quadriceps of that leg. With weak quadriceps the balance is maintained by arching or extending the lumbar spine, which can be painful. When the lift is larger, the effort required becomes much greater and the body mechanics become more complicated. When climbing on a high stool or chair, it should be done with the assistance of the hands on some external supporting structure. With a ladder the rails provide such assistance. With a chair or large stool there is no such assistance and the climb has to be achieved by body mechanics. The patient must lean forward over the object. This bend should occur from the hips and not the lumbar spine. The abdominal muscles should be tightened, and again good quadriceps muscles are required to push the patient up onto the lift. Coming down from such a large lift almost requires jumping. The balance and strength of the quadriceps required prohibits most patients from getting down in a forward position. Coming down backwards, as we do with ladders, uses easier body mechanics. The patient can also sit down on the higher lift and lower himself, taking advantage of the length of his legs, rather than having to jump and jolt the spine. Sliding forward off the lift from the sitting position can cause excessive extension of the lumbar spine and aggravation of a low back pain problem.

Sex

How soon after a back injury can a patient begin sexual activities? This again depends on the nature of the patient's back injury and the positions and activities that make him worse. Most sexual activity involves a pelvic tilt or thrust, which is actually one of the exercises that is taught early in the protection of the back. Vigorous pelvic thrusting, however, does cause the vertebral segment to pass through a considerable and sometimes even extreme range of motion. This can be damaging to a vertebral segment and certainly painful to the patient who already has problems.

Being a passive partner in the protected position by lying on the back in pelic tilt is generally very safe. Sidelying can also be safe. Generally speaking, most minor disc and facet injuries heal enough in a week or two to allow safe sexual activities. However, if there is a herniated disc with leg pain that is aggravated by even passive sexual activity, the patient should consider early diagnosis and treatment.

There is much emotion involved with sexual activities. The patient may either deny pain or use pain as an excuse. This is covered more thoroughly in the discussion on psychological problems in Chapter 4. The most significant information is that sex is rarely difficult, if a patient uses good body mechanics and has a good knowledge of sexual positions. These can be taught at the back school and for many come quite naturally.

Sex does not present a major problem with most back injuries, but dealing with a patient's emotions or getting him to change his usual sexual practices can be a big job for the back school.

Bed making

Making a bed is difficult for most patients with low back problems because beds are too low for most people's height. Making a bed reqires bending over for several minutes at a time, while lifting and pushing. Bending the knees is difficult when making a bed because bending the knees pushes a person away from the bed and he can no longer reach what he has to do. Therefore he has to bend over the bed with his knees fairly straight. This requires a good straight back hip bend. This position is tiring after a few minutes, so the patient bends his back while lifting, pushing, or twisting and injures the vertebral segment. As with most other solutions for back health care, if a patient becomes stronger, tightens his abdomen and his good endurance, the problem is solved.

The solution from a body mechanics point of view is to kneel down at the side of the bed and do the work directly in front of you. Kneeling down effectively shortens the individual to the level of the working space. It does eliminate the knees as a productive mechanism but being at the level of the work space eliminates the need for much back protection. The back can be straight, while the work is being done.

When the bed is large or the person is short, reaching far across the bed can be difficult and painful. From a standing position such a long reach requires considerable strength and balance to keep the back straight and the abdomen tight, while the knees are prevented from bending. From a kneeling position a person can learn or actually lie down on the bed as he reaches across to straighten a blanket or place a pillow. Of course kneeling takes more time and that again is a major problem in dealing with back pain patients. They are in a hurry just as everyone else. They are generally stressful and pressed for time. They need to be given stress management and to be convinced of the need to slow down their life-style so that they have time to practice good body mechanics.

Taking a shower

A shower can be a dangerous place, even for a person with a normal back. Surfaces are slick. The shower space is usually small and does not allow room for bending over comfortably. There are rarely good handles or supports to hold onto for protection. A straight backbend in a small cubicle shower is hardly possible because of the great deal of space necessary to do that particular bend. A simple squat is possible to pick up a bar of soap but vision is then obscured by the knees as the person lowers himself over the soap. There is also the problem of water in the face as the person attempts to squat. A good solution to some of these problems is a stool in the shower. A person can sit on a stool

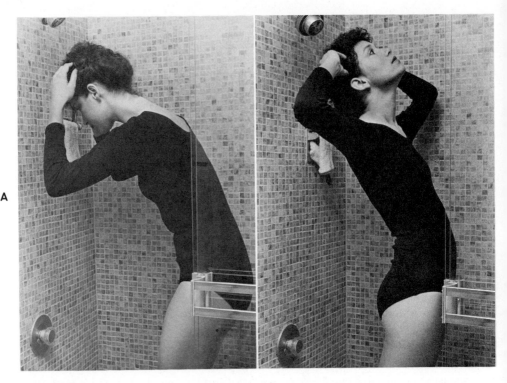

Fig. 6-27. Washing hair in the shower. **A**, Right: pelvic tilt, knees bent. **B**, Wrong: excess lumbar lordosis.

holding his abdomen tight and have better protection and support. A bar of soap on a string or a rope around the neck can be purchased or manufactured very easily. The patient can balance himself on the stool while washing his hair or stand facing the shower and then be directly in the flow of the water, rather than having to bend or arch to rinse the hair and other parts of the body (Fig. 6-27).

ERGONOMICS
Ergonomics of household activities

Ergonomics is the study of environmental situations to make them safer and more economical for energy expenditure and, in our particular field, for spinal protection. Thus there are changes that can be made in almost any situation to make it more appropriate for the patient's medical spinal condition as well as the avoidance of trauma to the spine. Many changes are not practical or possible, such as raising sinks to the appropriate level for the individual's height. A person kneels at the bedside to make the bed, rather than having one that is 5 feet high and difficult to get into. Placing a stool in a shower is a good ergonomics change for that particular activity. What other changes can we see in the ergonomics of household activities? The kitchen needs a lot of changes. Most kitchens have pots and pans either above or below working spaces. This requires a great amount of bending and reaching for frequently used items. Open shelving is one solution to this

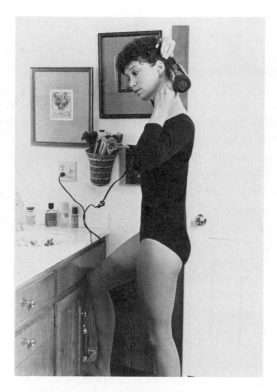

Fig. 6-28. Correct body mechanics for drying hair.

problem. Keeping frequently used items out on working spaces or hanging them at accessible heights is important. A simple analysis of the kitchen environment points out that rearrangement of the more frequently used items to the most easily accessible locations should be done first. While working at a sink for long periods of time, a foot should be up on a stool or lift. Various sized stools and lifts should be available. There are two- and three-level rolling stools made for kitchens that allow climbing to reach safely as well as supporting a leg to hold the body in pelvic tilt while ironing or doing bench and sink work. The cabinet door under a sink can be opened to allow elevation of foot (Fig. 6-28). Railings can be placed in frequently used standing areas. This is the reason that railings are placed at drinking bars. They allow the person to stand for long periods of time with one foot on the rail for resting the back. It seems quite interesting to me that the sinks in the kitchen are generally higher than sinks in the bathroom. Most people find that they have to bend over excessively at the sink in the bathroom to wash their face or brush their teeth. A kitchen sink allows these jobs to be done with a minimal amount of back bending.

Selection of equipment to be used around the house warrants some ergonomic expertise. In selecting your vacuum cleaner, for example, the shorter the working arm of the apparatus, the more bending a person naturally has to do. This needs to be balanced against the weight that needs to be pushed around. The large upright vacuum cleaners require considerable push and pull and present a difficult body mechanics problem. The smaller cannister models have a very light arm that does not require a lot of pushing and pulling even though the efficiency of the machine may not be as good. Here again the patient has to make some sacrifices in speed and efficiency for the protection of the spine. With the cannister model, however, there is more bending and lifting as one moves the cannister from place to place. There are of course major possibilities of changes in houses in which a centralized vacuum suction can be attached to each room so that there is no major equipment to be moved about for vacuuming. The base is simply plugged into whichever room needs to be vacuumed.

Placing chairs and stools of proper design in appropriate locations is one of the most valuable ergonomic changes that a person can make in his home. A stool at the kitchen and bathroom sinks allows a patient to sit while working or shaving. He can adjust their height to the countertop and lean on that with one elbow, while working with the other hand. Most kitchen chairs are not suited for back pain patients. Therefore seated work in the kitchen is usually not restful. A good chair with a slanted back and a work space that can be pulled to the patient can allow many hours of comfortable sitting work each day.

Toilets and bathroom spaces should be arranged to suit the back pain patient. Bending over first thing in the morning to raise a toilet seat before the spine adjusts to being in the erect position, can be painful and one of the beginning incidences of back trauma each day. The conventional level of toilet bowls is good for most people who have normal knees and hips. If the patient is unable to squat because of knee or hip pathology or weak quadriceps muscles, an elevated toilet seat can be obtained. The conventional level of the toilet bowl allows the patient to lean forward from the hips, resting his elbows on his knees. This prevents full lumbar flexion, as would otherwise be present if the patient simply relaxed and sagged forward to a conventional slumped sitting position. The patient can also support himself in a straight back position by holding onto the side of the toilet seat with his hands and extending his elbows.

The location of the toilet paper holder is frequently a ridiculous distance from the toilet. The patient has to twist, turn, and bend while sitting, which can be painful or damaging.

Straining during a bowel movement is painful for many low back patients. Attention to good diet and use of a stool softener can prevent much of this type of pain.

Clothes

Wearing apparel should be specialized for back pain patients. It is difficult to put on tights, narrow boots, or tight stockings. When a patient has to bend forward and stand on one foot to achieve some of these dressing assignments, the back is in great jeopardy. Squatting, sitting, or lying down to accomplish them is much safer (Fig. 6-29). The back should be stabilized against a wall (or a firm surface if lying down) while the hips and knees bring the feet as close to the patient's hands as possible. The wearing apparel can be altered in an ergonomic fashion to make dressing rapid and easy. Looser clothes do not require lots of contortion and force and are safer for the back than tight clothes that require lots of pulling, forcing, and bending.

Loafers that can be slipped on or slippers, which do not require bending over to pull

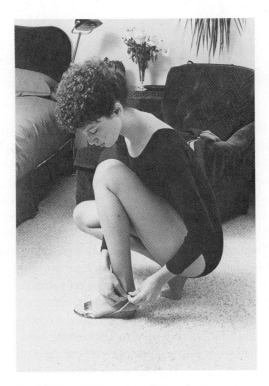

Fig. 6-29. Squatting to put on shoes.

on, are much better than boots and tie shoes. Of course they should not be so loose or sloppy that the patient is unstable on his feet. High heels throw the lumbar spine into more lordosis, and back pain patients frequently find an increase in their pain when they initially try to wear high-heeled shoes or boots. The stability of most high-heeled shoes is not as good as it is in flat shoes. This causes an increased strain on the back, and thus a simple change in shoe wear can reduce a back patient's pain. Wearing high-heeled shoes can cause a person to land heavier on the heels, causing a jarring action with every step. By bending the knees, much of that jarring ceases. Many patients with very high heels walk with their knees more flexed and rarely come into a full extended knee position.

Bathing

Bathtubs, hot tubs, and other such bathing pools are comfortable to most low back pain patients. Care must be taken in getting in and out especially of small tubs, which require fully flexed lumbar positions while lowering yourself into the tub. The slipperiness needs to be taken into account along with the strength and coordination of the individual. The protective handles and railings on tubs are generally better than they are in showers. Having a good grip with the hands and lowering yourself down slowly and safely to a sitting position is usually painless. Sitting in a tub for long periods of time, however, can result in full lumbar flexion as the individual sags forward. This can be prevented by supporting yourself with your hands or with a slanting back on the tub or seat. Brushes with handles allow the patient to get to his feet without having to lean far forward. A hand-held water sprayer or cup to pour water over the head and back can prevent some potentially dangerous contortions in a small tub.

REST PERIODS

The principle of adequate rest periods between working activities is very important for the newly active low back pain patient. A person does not always know how much damage he does to his spine during any particular activity. It seems to be human nature to take on more than you are capable of doing. Patients have a tendency to rapidly return to all of the things they were previously able to do, and they do them in an improper fashion, thus quickly causing them to return to an acute low back stage that requires bed rest again. Many even take pain medications to be able to do a day's work, only to have the medication wear off and find they are worse than they were before they started. This type of a cycle has to be broken. When a patient first becomes active, he should do one of the least strenuous, most simple household activities. Then he should rest for an hour or two in a contour position to be sure that there are no adverse effects (Fig. 6-30). He can then take on a slightly larger task. When the therapist finds that the patient is having pain after a particular activity or task, further investigation and training need to be done. Either the patient is doing the activity improperly or the patient's condition is not yet ready (and may never be ready) for that particular task. Further strengthening may be necessary. Greater understanding of the body mechanics for that particular task may be what is lacking.

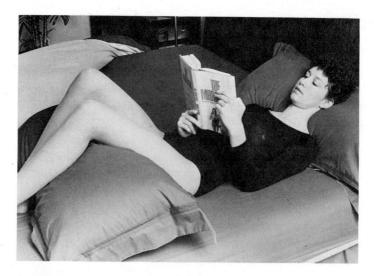

Fig. 6-30. Resting position.

PATIENT EVALUATION

There are innumerable variations of tasks, pathology, and body mechanics. For example, a patient with chronic facet disease who has arthritic knees is going to do vacuuming in a different way than a patient who has spinal stenosis and asthma. We have to take into consideration every one of these variations and help our patients adjust to them. This frequently requires simulating the task in the office for the patient or actually going to the patient's home or work space to help him with his problems. It is easy for a therapist or person with good knowledge of body mechanics to do the particular task required. We then have to evaluate the problems that the patient is having with that task, considering his back pathology and general physical capabilities. When taking that into account, we can usually show the patient how to achieve the desired goal. If it is impossible for the patient to achieve that goal, some other changes are necessary. Those changes involve either altering the patient's strength, knowledge, and coordination, or changing the environment and task to be achieved. It may be totally unreasonable for the patient to expect to perform certain tasks in his physical condition or with his pathological state. Mechanization and ergonomics may be necessary. There are vacuum cleaners that are self-propelled. There are many ways to hoist or elevate working areas to a more reasonable level. Power tools can save considerable low back strain. Various sized step ladders can make difficult spaces accessible.

Stresses and emotional tension in most patients' lives tend to sabotage their own best interests. The back pain patient who is attempting to care for her back while she is raising infants or trying to maintain a certain standard of living for her husband and family, the businessman who has deadlines to meet and trips to take, and the athlete with one more game that he absolutely must play are just a few of the situations in which we find a patient unwilling or unable to cooperate in his own care. Educating this type of patient in his own management is imperative. He must be taught that he has to take responsibility for his own pain and remain free of it. He may not use medication to keep going, and he must change his life-style and environment to fit his new back status. This type of education takes considerable time, patience, and many mistakes along the way. The basic back school, as presented in the previous chapters, is gauged at that average back pain patient without all the complications and problems. If it is difficult to convince the patient, it can sometimes take months of trial and error on his part before he is the master of his degenerative spine. If he is given the basic back school information but does not believe it or does not use it, he may continue to return to his doctor or therapist with the same complaints of pain, wanting something miraculous to take it away. He receives multiple treatments, including injections, braces, innumerable chiropractic treatments, and even surgery. Only an occasional fortunate patient is cured by any of these efforts for a significant period of time. If he does get some short-range relief, it is not long before he is back with complaints at the same or at a different level of his spine. He may go on for years before he finally accepts the changes that he has to make or before he simply develops new habit patterns in an automatic or reflex attempt to stay pain free.

Another individual who is very difficult to treat may be totally cooperative but society is demanding too much of him. He understands everything that you teach him and wants to cooperate fully, but his occupation demands more than is possible with a painful back. He has invested his entire working career in a particular job that is now too strenuous for him. Allowances have not been made by his employer or by our society to compensate for the new level of back capability. Being caught in a bind between employer's demands, financial stresses, and low back pain, a patient becomes emotionally distraught and begins to develop all kinds of secondary problems, which are more difficult than the back pain. The problems are discussed more thoroughly in Chapter 4. The physician and therapist need the assistance of many other paramedical specialists, including the rehabilitation consultant, the vocational consultant, psychologists, social workers, and frequently a whole team of various occupational and physical therapists, using back school and pain-control techniques.

7 BACK SCHOOL IN THE WORK ENVIRONMENT

The dilemma

The industrial back injury dilemma is a major problem for the industrial world. The problem of low back pain in industry is very complex and has four interrelated causes: lack of education, lack of communication, lack of interest, and lack of responsibility on the part of the individual worker, the employer, the industry, the union, the insurance compensation carrier, the medical profession, and the legal profession. These causes exist in various degrees.

The magnitude of the problem is almost unfathomable; we are talking of billions of dollars of expense each year in the United States alone. (In the United States in 1981 a conservative estimate of the cost of the industrial back dilemma was $1.9 billion.) The exact expense is difficult to determine because of the hidden dollar costs of insurance premiums, working days lost, decreased productivity, medical costs, and vocational rehabilitation training costs. This monetary expense is nothing when compared to the human and social suffering of individuals who have low back pain and are unable to continue working.

Some generalities for the magnitude of the problem can be made. More than 80% of the world's population is going to suffer some disabling low back pain in their lives. Over 70 million people in the United States visit the doctor's office annually, complaining of low back pain. Seventeen million of these people have recurrent back pain. Half of these people are between the ages of 21 and 45 years old, the working age group. The problem is essentially an epidemic.

Even though 90% of back pain episodes subside spontaneously, the circumstances that lead to the back pain, in most cases, do not change, so the back pain has a great likelihood of recurring. Ten percent of back pain episodes do not subside spontaneously, and those are the ones that cost billions of dollars and lead to the industrial back dilemma.

If we can prevent the original back injury, we have solved half of the problem. If we cannot prevent the initial injury, at least we can prevent the recurrent injury from becoming permanently disabling. With proper evaluation, treatment, education, and minor changes in the work environment, we can take all of the individuals with back injuries and return most of them to productive working activities with a minimum of time and expense through the use of the principles of back school.

To apply the back school principles to the work environment, we need to look at several aspects of the industrial back dilemma. Between 20% and 50% of injuries occurring in industry involve the low back. Some industries are subject to a tremendous potential back injury rate, either because of the nature of the work being done or the nature of the psychosocial factors surrounding that industry. The cost of industrial back injuries is almost twice that of other industrial injuries.

Back pain begins at 30 or 35 years of age on the average. This is a period of time in a working person's life when he is usually striving excessively and caring for his body minimally. Most individuals reach their peak physical condition in their late teens and early 20s. As they stop exercising and begin working, they gain weight and lose strength. As this deconditioning process continues, the individual's capability of performing a certain task decreases. Finally the individual's strength and body mechanics no longer protect him from injury and he begins having a multiplicity of musculoskeletal problems including tennis elbow, carpal tunnel syndrome, bursitis, arthritis, sprains, strains, and degenerative lumbar disc disease, all of which are the result of accumulated trauma. Since most individuals are spending a third of their time working, it is quite likely that the patient feels his back pain happened at work or is intensified by work. It is reported as an industrial injury and becomes part of the industrial back dilemma.

Along with the deconditioning process that goes on, there are the four previously stated causes for the industrial back dilemma: education, communication, disinterest, and responsibility.

We believe education could significantly reduce, if not totally eradicate, the industrial back dilemma immediately, as it has diseases such as tuberculosis and typhoid. It is simply a matter of low back hygiene, as it is with dental hygiene. We have learned from the diligent educational campaign by the dental profession that, if we properly take care of our teeth on a daily basis, we rarely have significant long-range problems. We need industrial as well as individual education for our backs but we also need to educate our children and our workers in low back health care. Keeping fit and working properly is all that is usually necessary for a person to avoid significant low back pain problems.

Industries such as Southern Pacific Transportation Companies and Safeway Stores, Inc., which have instituted educational programs, have decreased their back injuries 20% to 50%. Education is successful in decreasing costs for the care of diabetes, rheumatoid arthritis, hemophilia, and many other disease processes. As we apply educational principles to the industrial back dilemma through the use of back school, we are progressively solving the problem.

Communication is another major key to solving the industrial back dilemma. Communication is not good between workers and their supervisors, employers and insurance companies, insurance companies and unions, unions and management, physicians and their patients, or physicians and employers. Attorneys then become involved to support the patient in his communication. The insurance companies and industries become alarmed at the involvement of attorneys and thus communication is often further reduced. Through this lack of communication, we create the industrial back dilemma out of an otherwise reasonably simple, often curable, and certainly controllable back injury.

Disinterest is much of the reason for this lack of communication and education.

Industries have not realized the cause of the industrial back dilemma and therefore have not supported educational programs. Medicine has been preoccupied with more serious problems, such as cancer and heart disease. Through heavy efforts of various societies such as Easter Seals, many other major diseases have been virtually eradicated. There has not been this great interest in back pain. There has never been an official specialty in medicine devoting itself to low back pain. It was not until the early 1970s that orthopaedic surgeons began subspecializing in back pain. In dealing intensively with the industrial back dilemma for the past 10 years, I have yet to be able to interest any union organization in entering into back education and prevention programs. We have, however, interested an increasing number of industries and insurance companies in providing back health care and education to their employees.

Ultimately the industrial back dilemma boils down to responsibility. No one wants to take the responsibility for low back pain. The injured worker, naturally, does not want the responsibility because he can no longer support himself and pay for his medical bills. He does not understand what the back injury means and has enumerable fears and problems. The employer does not want the cost of the injury, much less the cost of having to educate the employees who should have had the education before they came into the industry. Society has not taken on the responsibility of public education in schools and on television as it has with dental hygiene and other illnesses. Medicine has begun to take on some responsibility but is moving very slowly at this time. Insurance companies, having to bear much of the cost of the industrial back dilemma, have been forced to take on the responsibility of some education, training, and research. The professionals who have shown the most interest and responsibility for the industrial back dilemma to date are the people running back schools.

The solution

The back school can spearhead the solutions for the industrial back dilemma. Eventually back schools will be part of all public education and all industrial training, safety, and retraining programs. For now the back school professionals must take the lead. The subsequent discussion involves the current solution to the industrial back dilemma as recommended from the back school concept.

PREVENTION OF BACK INJURIES

Workers must be selected for a particular job. Despite the complaints from unions, attorneys, and civil rights groups, it is not safe or reasonable to have a deconditioned, weak, or untrained person do heavy back labor. We have enough problems keeping strong, healthy, trained people from injuring their backs, much less forcing industry to start out with workers who are certain to be injured. You would not expect an industry to hire a secretary who could not type. It is equally ridiculous to hire a laborer who cannot lift and bend safely. Back school professionals need to work closely with industry and other professionals to help set some guidelines.

Management in industry must be convinced to select the worker and then train him to protect himself for the particular job he is doing. Back school can do this training. Each job must be analyzed for its potential of creating back injury. Each employee must be instructed in the potential for back injury and trained to do the job so that the likelihood of him having a back injury is much less. Thus the worker is given some choice and responsibility in the matter. He knows the risks and the requirements. If he falls below a certain level of strength, endurance, coordination, or willingness to perform the task properly, he knows that he is creating his own back problems. With training we can give the worker the necessary education so that he can take responsibility for his action and is more likely to affect the consequences. In addition the management knows that it has provided an opportunity for those who are willing to accept responsibility.

Management must be willing to look at the tasks that need to be performed and realistically decide who is able to do them. Those jobs with high risk of injury need to be changed. It is quite unreasonable to expect most human beings to lift 100-pound sacks for 20 or 30 years. By the time most of us are approaching the 60-year-old mark, we are not in condition to continue this kind of work. Therefore jobs need to be either mechanized or employees need to be transferred from certain jobs. This leads us to one of the major changes that some of the more enlightened industries are making. They are providing alternative jobs for each employee. There is one heavy job and one light job. If they find that for some reason and at some time in the worker's career, he is unable to continue his job, they have the other one for which the employee has been gradually trained and can change over without a great deal of expense, retraining, or industrial back dilemma conflict. The back school, through its knowledge of ergonomics, can help industry look at these jobs and employees and can help decide what types of work are reasonable and what alternatives are available. This applies at both the prevention and return-to-work levels.

There needs to be ongoing reinforcement for all employees. It is human nature to forget or become lazy and return to old, improper styles of lifting and bending. Reminders can be provided in various forms of posters, classes, contests, and verbal reminders, such as Safeway has provided in its professional weight-lifter back prevention program.

This brings us to the general fitness or well-being programs that are being instituted in some industries. This is usually done for the "more valuable" employees in higher management. There have long been annual complete physical evaluations and rest and relaxation programs ordered for the high-tension businessman. Education and provisions for all employees to have good overall health are necessary. Such programs can be provided by anything as extensive as a gymnasium or recreation center associated with a particular plant or factory. Classes in general health, stress management, the meaning of well-being, and the importance of the aging process can be provided on a regular basis to employees and even the families of employees. Back education is simply part of this overall health, education, and training. Organizations such as the YMCA have these types of programs on a regular basis.

MANAGEMENT OF BACK INJURIES

We cannot expect to eliminate all injuries; therefore if an accident occurs and the employee has a back injury, several changes must be made. The reporting of the injury has long been inadequate. The patient does not think anything of the injury at first and goes home but the next day he cannot get out of bed. He does not remember the incident. In some cases when he reports it the following day, the employer feels the worker had the accident at home but wants to blame it on his job. Education of both the employer and employee in how these kinds of conflicts develop improves the reporting of the accident. It also allows immediate medical care rather than having an employee try to soldier on for many months with a back injury that is a mystery to him and gets worse and worse and may become irreparable.

The employer or industry must investigate all injuries more extensively. How many similar types of injuries have occurred? Is there something about this particular job or task that needs to be changed? Are there certain qualifications of employees that would better fit this particular task?

The injured employee also needs good medical care. In the past he has been sent to the closest, fastest, cheapest industrial clinic. Back schools need to be included in these local industrial clinics. The clinic physicians need to be trained with regard to the true nature of back injuries. They have been calling all back injuries "back sprains" for decades. These sprains almost always herald some underlying and ongoing degenerative segment process. They must not continue to play down the back injury and send the patient back to the bad habits and mistakes that brought him there in the first place. A serious look must be taken at every employee who has a back injury. His body mechanics and strengths must be evaluated. His knowledge of the job and the body mechanics necessary must be evaluated. Remedial back school should be given. If the injured worker does not respond rapidly to good care locally, he should be referred to a very knowledgeable spinal specialist who rapidly and economically evaluates the patient, trains him further, and comes to a conclusion that is accepted by the worker, industry, and insurance carriers.

Too often the injured worker chooses his own doctor, whereas the insurance company chooses another doctor. There is conflict in opinion as to what is wrong. The worker becomes confused, and much time is wasted. The employer replaces the injured worker, who hires an attorney, and we are back to the industrial back dilemma. There is a very well-accepted timetable of events and a general treatment and evaluation plan that can be followed by any physician who is interested in back pain. If this timetable is accepted by all participants in the industrial back dilemma, the confusion, frustration, and expense can all be avoided.

Communication among all of the members of the team is extremely important. Reports and telephone calls must be made quickly between the industrial clinic, the specialist's office, the industrial nurse, the employer, and the personnel offices. The back school can provide this intermediary communication. The back school professional teaches the injured employee what is wrong. The treatment plan is outlined for the patient as well as the employer. The physician is saved much of the time of teaching and communicating. If the patient is not improving as anticipated, the back school immediately has him return to the physician for further diagnostic tests and communication with the industry.

The industry must be willing to train its health nurses and safety personnel in back school methods. The entire back school can be given within the industry itself. Thus the industry is managing its own back injuries with some guidance from the local physicians. If this is not possible, at least the safety instructors are acutely aware of body mechanics and back health care. They are observing their fellow employees on a regular basis.

The best success in back prevention has been seen at the Southern Pacific Transportation Companies. The key to its success was training fellow workers to deliver the back school. The trainers were co-workers at Southern Pacific and spoke the same language. They were generally well-liked and respected by the other workers. Employees often accept the education and recommendations much better from these types of individuals than from strangers who come from entirely foreign perspectives. To carry this concept even further, industries can provide a local counselor who helps fellow employees with things like "job burnout," overbearing or unsupportive supervisors, faulty equipment, or drug and alcohol problems. Employees are sometimes under heavy external and emotional stresses that make them more susceptible to back injuries. If these can be identified and the employee directed to adequate help early, much of the industrial back dilemma can be avoided. There are health organizations that provide form of support to any given industry. They provide newsletters, medical counselors, telephone advisement centers, and many other ongoing general health benefits.

Some insurance companies have encouraged the development of back care programs, giving rebates to industries that institute some of the previously mentioned changes in their policies and methods of dealing with back problems. Unions must not only stop dragging their feet, but actively participate in the preceding recommendations by providing much of the education, becoming the advocate of the patient, and assisting with communication.

You can see from the previous discussion that there are innumerable changes that can be made from any segment responsible for the industrial back dilemma. The back school acts as a catalyst to get these individuals participating.

Because of resistance in geographical areas or the local social structure and availability of specialists in the various organizations, the back school needs to lean more heavily on one group than another for assistance. If there is total cooperation by the industry, there are certain guidelines that we use in back school to help evaluate physical stressors in the work environment and to design the work task and work enviornment to minimize the risk of spinal injury. The remainder of this chapter concentrates on these specific changes. These thoughts are not intended as a treatise on ergonomics and work place design but as general guidelines to consider when analyzing or modifying the work environment.

Guidelines to work task and work environment design to minimize risk of spinal injury

History and statistical research show that present employee selection techniques and general instruction concerning safe lifting as previously applied has not been effective in reducing or controlling material handling and, specifically, spinal injuries. Better selection with appropriate physical tests for the particular job and specific job-related training should improve the picture.

A more recent and effective approach is to design stress-producing factors out of the work task and the work environment. With good design the worker is exposed to less stress regardless of his physical condition or adherence to rules of good body mechanics.

Work task and environmental design changes in combination with new methods of teaching and motivating safe employee body mechanics appear to be the most reasonable and logical approach to the back injury problem. Strength testing, exercise, and nutrition also have their place, but they are less controlled and measured.

Many factors that bear on the back injury problem for industry include characteristics of the worker, material being handled, task design, and work environment. To establish an effective safety program, each level of involvement must take responsibility for those elements that are under its influence and control. As a generalization, we might assign the elements in this manner:

The *employee* learns to adjust his work area for optimum ergonomic design. He learns to use good material handling techniques and to work at prescribed rates to avoid fatigue. He needs to inform the supervisor of areas that appear to have either potential or already existing problems.

The *employer* has the responsibility of learning and becoming aware of good work task and work environment design. A safety officer or supervisor should be trained. Supervisors encourage and help ensure the use of proper body mechanics by their employees. They must also apply a motivational manner to improve compliance.

The *safety officer* is expected to know good body mechanics and guidelines for work task and environmental design. He assists supervisors in the analysis of job tasks and their work environments. Back school can train the safety officer, the supervisors, and employees in proper body mechanics. The program is better managed by the training of supervisors or other ky personnel in motivation and compliance techniques. This training is completed by the safety officer often in conjunction with another professional such as the company occupational health nurse, the registered nurse, or an outside consultant. Educational and training programs need to be tailored specifically for each industry and at times even for specific segments of an industry. The information needs to be simple and presented in a style acceptable to the employee. The information should be stimulating, entertaining, and capable of holding the attention of those being trained.

Management must be actively involved and careful not to put the majority of the responsibility for safety on the supervisors, employees, or safety officer. It is beneficial to be aware of the factors that affect your employees in both production and safety; look further than the mechanical task; watch for social and environmental factors. It is then important to apply this knowledge to the processes, rates, and equipment, as well as to the employees.

The following sections contain information and guidelines for lifting, carrying, pushing, and pulling. Seated and standing operators and truck drivers are considered separately. No matter what our level of knowledge, the major elements needed to prevent injuries are (1) good job analysis, (2) willingness to make changes, and (3) involvement with employees.

LIFTING

Lifting has been identified by almost everyone as a major source of back injuries. In an in-depth study by Dr. Stover Snook of Liberty Mutual, regarding its policyholders, it was found that 70% of all lost-time injuries are related to material handling. Of this 70%, 55% was directly related to lifting. This means that 38.5% of all lost-time injuries over the period studied was directly related to lifting. Other researchers and statisticians have published figures that indicate the injurious effect of lifting and other material handling is in the range of 25% to 50% of all lost-time injuries. Twenty-five percent of the Liberty Mutual policyholders had a majority of manual handling tasks requiring strength and endurance factors found in less than 25% of the general working population. Tasks that are not acceptable to 75% of the work population show an injury rate three times higher than those that fall within the 75% guidelines.

Object factor guidelines

When lifting heavy objects, the need for manual lifting should be minimized whenever possible by the use of good work place design and lifting aides, such as conveyors (powered and gravity fed), hoists and cranes, hydraulic lift hand trucks, skids and pry bars, and team lifting techniques. Weights should be lifted within the limits acceptable to 75% of the working population and consideration should be given to the difference between male and female workers. Values are available from the National Institute of Occupational Safety and Health (NIOSH).

The container size should be as small as possible with the primary concern being the horizontal distance from the body. Containers should be purchased with dimensional limitations in mind. They should be avoided when they have dimensions that cause the worker to have his arms more than 30 degrees to the front or side. A good general rule is to limit the width dimension to 20 inches and the length to 28 inches. It is also important to keep the load balanced so that the worker does not have to apply forces to control a moving center of gravity or to stabilize an asymmetrical load.

Handles can increase the grip strength of the worker and reduce the chance of losing control. Rough textured surfaces tend to be easier to grip than smooth ones. Poorly fitting gloves or soiled gloves can inhibit the grip and be a disadvantage to the worker; they should fit well and be in good condition.

Technique factor guidelines

Proper lifting techniques require the load to be kept close and the intraabdominal pressure high. Situations such as cluttered areas that require the worker to reach over another object to lift should be excluded from the design. Good lifting techniques should be taught and monitored so that the proper methods become a habit. Work stations should be designed so that the work heights do not encourage poor techniques. Loads more than 20 inches from the body severely increase stress, and loads more than 40 inches away are intolerable for most workers.

High-frequency lifting from low levels is to be avoided. It takes more energy to use the conventional straight back, bent knee method of lifting, which increases fatigue and subsequently encourages poor technique.

The worker should absolutely eliminate the combination of twisting and lifting. He needs to lift either straight ahead or at a diagonal stance. If he must move to the side with or without an external load, he should turn his feet, not his torso. If at all possible, equipment should be turned rather than people, which can be accomplished by strategic placement of pallets, control of roller or conveyor line direction, knowledge of loading procedures and sequences, and placement of stops and shut-offs within reach so that twisting is not necessary. If twisting cannot possibly be eliminated, it must be minimized.

Smooth, well-coordinated movement is to be encouraged. Sequential tasks that require quick starts and stops or abrupt changes in height or direction should be reduced or eliminated. Tasks that use muscle activity as a substitute for mechanical stops should not be designed.

Lifting should not start from below knee height, so the design should originate around tall workers. Similarities and differences among workers should be known. NIOSH suggests that women generally lift 70% of male values for weight and distance. In mixed areas, the design should be geared toward the 75% female value, not the 75% male value. Both male and female workers are able to lift more weight at low frequency, such as one lift or less per minute, especially from ground to knuckle height. In high frequency lifting (three or more lifts per minute), men lift more between knuckle and shoulder height, whereas women do not show significant variations in lifting from floor to knuckle and knuckle to shoulder. Both male and female workers can lift less from shoulder to reach height. Work should be below shoulder height, if possible, with 50 inches being the maximum work height. Therefore these heights should be designed around shorter workers. It is important to note that both males and females can lower more weight than they can lift. The vertical distance lifted should be minimized. On- and off-loading heights should match; platforms should be used; spring-loaded pallet platforms are often valuable. Lifting should begin at approximately the shortest workers' knuckle heights.

Work load equals foot-pounds per minute. This is different from object weight. Research indicates that work load rates are maximum at one lift every 5 to 10 seconds. It is often necessary to adjust the rate to account for the variation in object factors such as weight and size. People working at high work loads should be allowed more frequent work breaks, as light weights at high repetitions can be very fatiguing. A maximum heart rate of 115 to 120 beats per minute has been recommended by some as a good guideline for conditioned male and female employees working at high rates.*

HEAT STRESS AND OTHER ENVIRONMENTAL CONSIDERATIONS

Heat stress can account for a 10% to 20% reduction in tolerated weights. More frequent breaks should be allowed for workers in hot areas; air conditioning and fans should be used whenever possible; workers should be rotated; humidity needs to be controlled; and rates should be adjusted to take heat stress into account.

There are other environmental considerations to be minimized. Noise is a distraction

---

*Based primarily on the work of Stover Snook. The tote boxes used in his research did not require workers to lift with hands at floor level. The remainder of the section is a synthesis of materials from several researchers and relates to other activities in addition to lifting.

that can cause a lack of concentration. Cold contributes to muscle stiffness and requires more energy to hold normal body temperature. Body dehydration also occurs in the cold. Air contaminants affect breathing and oxygen intake and promote fatigue. Air contaminants sometimes cause hay fever or asthma, which also promotes fatigue. Poor lighting affects vision, causes psychological problems, and decreases the workers' perception of personal safety.

SOCIAL AND EMOTIONAL FACTORS

Industry must consider social and emotional factors affecting employees. An individual's attitude and cooperation toward work mates and supervisors can affect his productivity and safety. A worker's emotional state on and off the job; his job satisfaction and feeling of reward; as well as changes made in his hours, shifts, and working environment contribute to his control, his feeling of well-being, and his productivity at work. Attention must be paid to the general design and desirability of the work place as a factor in a worker's attitude toward his job.

EMPLOYEE PHYSICAL CONDITION GUIDELINES

Consideration should be given to physical examinations before employment, endurance testing, obstacle course, low back x-ray films, medical histories, and weight as an indicator of strength when considering new workers. These factors, however, should not be the sole criteria for hiring or not hiring an employee. Intraabdominal pressure measurements may be the ultimate test to give before employment.

If you are going to consider strength testing as part of the selection process, know what muscles are necessary in the work task. Several methods focusing on isometric back muscle strength have been suggested by different researchers but are probably better left to major research centers. The most well-known and quoted results have been published by Donald Chaffin from the University of Michigan, establishing strength requirements that are statistically validated.

It may be useful to develop a test for endurance and to base general strength testing on the actual job to be performed. In any case it is vital to encourage physical fitness and good nutrition among all employees. You can help in their endeavors by providing resources on mental and physical health.

CARRYING

There is an element of carrying in every job we do. Often the industrial worker must carry the load once it has been lifted. Carrying activities should be kept to a minimum. Both males and females can lift much more than they can carry, even if the frequency is only once a day. Greater loads can be carried at knuckle height than at elbow height.

Objects being carried should not cause forward flexion of the trunk or abduction of the arms greater than 30 degrees. With arm abduction angles greater than 30 degrees, the shoulder muscles do not work effectively, which causes fatigue and increased back stress.

Loads should not be carried up steps, if at all possible, because vision is often blocked, loss of footing is more likely, and walking up steps requires increased energy expenditure as the legs must lift the body and the load an additional distance.

Balance and good footing need to be encouraged by keeping areas clear so that the worker has room to move. Objects need to be kept out of aisles and walking surfaces should be kept free of water, oil, dust particles, etc., to minimize slipping. Bulky loads can restrict vision and increase the chances of losing control, so mechanical aids or team carrying should be used with large loads whether they are light or heavy.

Lateral bending at approximately shoulder width needs to be eliminated or mini- mized. Controls should be within easy reach and loads should be carried on the shoulder rather than at the side, if appropriate. Half the load should be carried in each hand to balance the sides, if it is safe, and the worker should be careful of asymmetrical loads. Two people should be used whenever possible, if the object is awkward to carry. Carrying may be circumvented by using powered conveyors, realigning the work station, and using other power lifting and carrying equipment. When the frequency of carrying changes, adjustments must be made in the weights carried or other factors must be changed to compensate for the increased work load. Based on the work load (foot-pounds per minute) concept, maximum acceptable work load generally occurs in carrying with higher frequency rates and lighter loads. No specific fatigue studies have been completed, but the following appears to be a good compromise between work load and fatigue:

1. One 2.1 m carry every 12 to 15 seconds
2. One 4.3 m carry every 20 to 30 seconds
3. One 8.5 m carry every 30 to 60 seconds

These recommendations may be a little conservative, but it is better to err on the side of safety.

PUSHING AND PULLING

Pushing and pulling join with lifting and carrying to complete the major dynamic manual handling activities found in industry. As with lifting and carrying, there are a number of controllable factors that affect the ability of the worker to perform safely.

Females are able to push 75% to 80% of the male capacity for both initial and sustained pushing forces. There is a significant difference, 50% to 100%, in the ability of both males and females to exert initial push force and their ability to sustain that force. Care must be taken to ensure that initial force requirements do not exceed acceptable levels, even if the secondary sustained force requirements are acceptable. Carts with worn wheels on bad bearings that are pushed on softer surfaces require much greater initial force. Carts with new wheels and good bearings that are rolled on hard surfaces require less force.

It seems best for men and women to push at a height approximately midway between knuckle and elbow. Both males and females are able to generate greater initial forces at such a height than at shoulder height or below knuckle height. The sustained forces are generally the same at all levels.

Pushing should be kept to a minimum distance because the acceptable initial and sustained forces cause fatigue with increased distance. Weights must be lessened the more frequent the push, no matter what the distance, and pushing should be used instead of pulling whenever possible.

Effective pushing depends on good traction. The type of floor surface and shoe sole are critical. The best all-purpose floor surfaces are rubber pad, rubber tile, wood (soft and grain), rough concrete, linoleum, vinyl tile (smooth), and vinyl asbestos tile (smooth). The best all-purpose shoe soles are rubber cork soles, flat and dry; UAA-USAF standard sole, dry; rubber crepe sole, flat and dry; rubber overshoe, dry; neoprene, flat and dry; and leather, also flat and dry.

The worker needs to be aware of certain pitfalls. He should know that body weight is not a good predictor of strength; that tall persons tend to underestimate their maximum force; and that short persons tend to overestimate their maximum force.

The worker should avoid pushing and pulling in cramped or confined spaces or any time the body is in a vulnerable configuration. He should push and pull in line with the body. The cross-body push is the strongest with the body in a diagonal plane. This means there is slight rotation of the trunk in relationship to the load, but not any rotation between shoulders and hips. In a sideways push there is less strength, less balance, and more chance for injury. He should not push or pull with the body in one plane and the legs facing another plane because this causes severe twisting or rotation of the spine and increases torsional stress on the back. He needs to set his abdominal muscles, and use good body mechanics. Finally he needs to remember to push using his legs rather than his arms whenever it is possible.

SEATED AND STANDING OPERATORS

Poor design of equipment or work station layout induces stressful working postures in both the seated and the standing worker. Poor posture ultimately leads to fatigue, inefficiency, and reduced output, and to accidents or cumulative injury. In a study at Kodak, sedentary workers suffered only 12% less than standing workers, according to reports of back pain.

The actual size, location, and orientation of the work area for both the standing and seated operator are ultimately affected by the size of the work piece, the classification of work (precision, light, heavy), the motions required to accomplish tasks, the forces needed to accomplish the task, and the equipment used in the work place.

In general, sitting is preferable to standing because sitting requires less overall muscle activity to maintain posture. there is less intramuscular pressure in the lower extremities, which is a condition that is considered critical, especially for female workers. In upright sitting without proper support, however, the load on the L3 disc can be 43% greater than in a standing position.

Sitting position

A sitting position is indicated when stable posture is needed for tasks that require precise or fine movements; when the operator is required to operate foot controls; and when the choice is between extended sitting or extended standing work.

When provided a work space for the seated operator, there are specific areas that need attention. Seated worker body dimensions vary depending on the height and sex of the worker.

Work surface height. The work station should also be designed for the standing operator. If the work station is used for sitting and standing operators, the work height should be designed for the standing operator with the chair (stool) selection accommodating the seated position.* Ayoub makes recommendations in *Human Factors* with regard to sitting. The raised surfaces for fine assembly and precision work account for the better visual acuity required. If magnifiers or microscopes are used, these raised work surfaces may not be necessary. If magnifiers and microscopic work is ongoing, the worker's trunk position and trunk height must be taken into account and an adjustable chair or stool provided.

Work surface inclination. Often it is possible to incline the work surface. A 10-degree inclination serves to reduce the amount of neck flexion, which reduces cervical and upper thoracic stress. This also eliminates forward leaning, which increases low back stress.

Work space. To accommodate seated workers, whether they are at a desk, work bench, conveyor line, or assembly area, the work space must allow for sufficient leg and arm room.

Leg room
1. Minimum width 20 inches
2. Depth 25 inches, if limited
Work area
1. Four inches from edge of work surface
2. At least 100 square inches symmetrical to the worker, approximately 10 × 10 inches
Work height
1. 26 inches minimum for knee clearance

If these dimensions are not available, alterations are necessary. As a general rule, the work surface height should be at the elbow or slightly above.

Chair. The chair or work stool is the seated worker's interface with his environment. It is a tool, and therefore it is essential that proper consideration be given to this element of the work station. A proper work chair should have specific features.

Good lumbar (low back) support. Good lumbar support reduces intradiscal pressure and compensatory activity in posterior paraspinal muscles and should be height adjustable to begin at the worker's belt line.

Height adjustment. Height adjustment accommodates variations in worker dimensions, work station height, and work task to minimize the forward leaning of the worker and to minimize neck flexion. The elbow angle should be 90 degrees when the chair is adjusted for the work surface. A foot stool may be necessary.

Movement in the back support. Movement keeps the spine dynamic. Reclining reduces disc pressure by transferring part of the body weight to the chair back. Ten to 20 degrees of reclining is often quoted as satisfactory.

Foot support. Foot and leg contact with the floor gives the trunk and pelvic muscles a base of support against which to work. If the feet do not touch the floor, a foot rest is

---

*Ayoub, M.M.: Human factors, pp. 265-268, 1973.

required to keep the pelvis properly aligned (knees at or above hip level) and to reduce posterior thigh pressure, which can restrict blood circulation and cause swelling of the feet and ankles as well as numbness and tingling symptoms.

Seat angulation. A properly angulated seat keeps the hips flexed at 105 degrees, tips the pelvis forward and induces normal lumbar lordosis (curvature), does not overstretch the muscles and ligaments of the low back, and has sufficient friction between the seat and the worker, which prevents sliding forward.

Controls. Foot pedals should not require leg pumping action. The heel should remain on the ground, if possible. The line of action of the foot when activating the control or pedal should be directly through the hip. Stops and shutoffs should be within easy reach and should not require side or forward leaning, twisting, bending, or quick abrupt movements to operate.

Standing position

A standing position is indicated when large forces are needed, when larger spaces need to be covered, and when the work place is designed to alternate between sitting and standing. When providing a work space for the standing operator, there are also specific areas that need attention.

Standing worker's body dimensions. The elbow height above the floor is the critical dimesion for the standing worker and is approximately 45 inches for men and 42.5 inches for women.

Work surface height. Work surface height is generally 2 to 4 inches below elbow height when performing manual work. This makes a good working surface height 41 to 43 inches for men and 38.5 to 40.5 inches for women in the standing position.

Work space. Work space must be sufficient for knees and feet, which is approximately 6 inches at a minimum. There should be room for a footrest 6 to 10 inches to induce the "bar rail" pelvic tilt position. Extra room should be available based on the seated operator, if the work station is to be suitable for both seated and standing work. There should be room for the worker to move about at will and change position easily.

Work surface inclination. It is desirable, if possible, to incline the work surface approximately 10 degrees to reduce the neck flexion, which lessens the stress on the cervical and upper thoracic spine.

Controls. Foot pedals are not advised for the standing operator because it causes asymmetry in the muscle pattern, uneven mechanical stresses on the spine, and higher potential for slipping or losing balance. If foot pedals must be used, they should be operable with either foot. Stops, guards, and limit switches should be within easy reach and should not require side or forward leaning, twisting, bending, or quick abrupt movements to operate.

Other considerations. There should be a shock-absorbing surface on which to stand, such as a rubber mat or plywood platform. Shoes should be comfortable, supportive, and shock absorbing. Shoes with heels higher than 1 inch should be avoided. Work breaks that are more frequent than union requirements can have physical and mental benefits, especially for strenuous or tedious tasks.

TRUCK DRIVING

Persons who spend more than half their working hours driving are three times more likely to develop back problems than the average worker. This fact has been attributed to the following reasons:

- They sit for prolonged periods with poor back support.
- After prolonged sitting, they may immediately begin work (lifting, carrying, pushing, pulling) that varies from light to heavy.
- Sitting for prolonged periods with legs extended fatigues leg, hip, and back muscles.
- They experience constant vibration in the 2 to 15 Hz range. The 4 to 8 Hz range has been sown to be harmful to the discs, with 16 Hz affecting the head mostly, 32 Hz the lower body, and 64 Hz the ischial tuberosities.
- Many who use soft seat cushions actually are increasing the vibration effects.
- They experience forces related to starting and stopping a vehicle.
- Manual steering induces axial torques because of the push-pull forces on the horizontal wheel.
- Manual steering wheels often require forward leaning to operate because of their horizontal orientation.
- Most pedals require frequent leg lifting to operate, and the leg muscles operate in a biomechanically inefficient manner.
- Bouncing in the seat requires trunk muscle activity to stabilize the torso.

Recommended guidelines to reduce low back stress in truck drivers (also applies to equipment operators, such as forklift, backhoe, and caterpillar)

Minimize postural stress. To minimize postural stress, the seat back should be in a 15- to 20-degree reclining position. It should be at approximately a 6-degree backward tilt. The low back needs to be supported with the apex at L3 (on belt line), using a well-designed seat, seat insert (Sacro-Ease), or small pillow. These reduce flexion torques of the spine and psoas muscle (hip) activity and distribute acceleration forces over the back rest. The hip angle should be 105 degrees.

Minimize muscle effort. Muscle effort may be minimized by using power steering to reduce spinal stresses caused by the axial torque necessary for push-pull steering and the forward lean of a normal steering position. Pedals should be operated with the heel on the floor whenever possible and with the line of action through the foot to the hip rather than in a vertical direction. This maximizes muscle efficiency and reduces spinal stresses, assuming there is back support. This may not be entirely possible in existing equipment, but should be considered in future purchases.

Use seat belts. Seat belts and a shoulder harness or other trunk support should be used to minimize the muscle activity required to stabilize the upper body during bouncing and turning movements.

Minimize vibration effects. Vibration effects in a 4 to 8 Hz range should be minimized.

Firm cushions that do not bottom out over bumps and shock-absorbing seats that isolate the driver from the road vibration should be used.

Encourage exercise. The driver or operator should warm up slowly for about 5 minutes after sitting for more than 30 minutes, to stretch muscles and stimulate circulation. The minimum warm-up is leaning backward slowly 10 times after exiting from the truck or equipment. He should take a break from driving every 1 to 2 hours to help reduce the effects of vibration related to disc creep.

8 ATHLETIC BACK SCHOOL

Most back patients have questions regarding what athletic activities they can do and how they should do them. Such information is given in the basic back school's three sessions. There are many patients, however, who want to participate in a particular sport (or sports) and are willing to take considerable extra training to do so. Some are professional athletes but most are amateur athletes who have become so involved in their particular recreational sport that there is a surprising amount of emotional involvement. They would do anything, including having back surgery, to continue their sport. We can give these individuals an understanding of their medical spinal disorder and a general idea of the level of athletic activity at which they can participate with training. It is then their decision as to how extensively they are willing to train to accomplish their potential.

ATHLETICS AND SEVERITY OF SYMPTOMS

The sports or athletics that an individual with a bad back can participate in are related to the diagnosis and severity of the disease (Table 8-1).

Severe pain and disability

The individual with a herniated disc that gives him almost continual pain and that increases with almost all activities has the most difficult problem. It is similar to the individual with severe spinal stenosis, active ankylosing spondylitis, and some severe forms of degenerative disc and facet disease. These patients can do the basic isometric exercises that all of our patients are requested to do. These include isometric abdominal, gluteal, and quadriceps exercises. Once these muscle groups are maximally developed

Table 8-1. Potential athletic capabilities by diagnosis

Diagnosis	Physical strength and condition	Athletic capabilities
Severe abnormality	Poor	Bed rest
	Good	Swimming, bicycling, skiing, bowling
	Excellent	Doubles tennis, jogging, baseball
Mild abnormality	Poor	Swimming, bicycling, skiing, bowling
	Good	Jogging, tennis, baseball
	Excellent	All sports except contact and out-of-control sports

and the patient understands and uses excellent body mechanics, he can do other athletic endeavors.

A person can do weight lifting by positioning himself against a wall in a pelvic tilt position, holding himself with his abdominals and quadriceps while he works on the muscles of his upper extremities (Fig. 8-1, *A*). He can also lie on a bench in a knee- and hip-flexed position doing bench presses (Fig. 8-1, *B*). Other calisthenics and gymnastics can be similarly accomplished. Push-ups can be done with a very flat back and tightly held abdomen. Hanging exercises, both by the arms or by the legs, give traction on the vertebral segments while the exercises are being performed. The gravitonics gym is a device that can be hung in doorway to accomplish these exercises under gravity traction. Other stationary sports activities that allow the back to be put in a safe position and held there while the arms, legs, eyes, and ears do the rest of the work are naturally achievable. These include such things as fishing, hunting, boating, sports car driving, flying, bicycling, and most spectator sports. In all of these the participant can learn to position himself standing, leaning, lying down, or sitting to keep his pain under control during the activity.

Swimming is a good exercise, if the person is a good swimmer and can control his body mechanics in the water. The buoyancy and the decreased forces on the spine and the horizontal rather than vertical position of the spine can be quite advantageous. Warm water feels good to most patients. Floats can be used to position the trunk while exercising the extremities.

Many patients become weakened by long-term illness and gain weight. This frequently requires participation in an active rehabilitation program of muscle strengthening so that they can enjoy exercise and recreation again.

Moderately disabled and painful

Patients who are moderately disabled and who have moderate pain experience pain almost every day, but not just with simple changes in position and activities. The pain comes on with repeated mildly abusive activities, such as jogging, horseback riding, long periods of sitting in bad seats (auditoriums), working with repeated bending and lifting, and generally poor body mechanics and back health care. The conditions that lead to this type of pain are the chronic phases of degenerative disc disease before they become herniated discs, facet arthritis, early spinal stenosis, mild to moderate ankylosing spondylitis, and small central herniated discs. The maximum that these individuals can accomplish in athletics is almost the average normal. Although they cannot be strong athletes and participate competitively very well, they are, however, able to accomplish almost every sport and athletic endeavor to some extent. The intensity to which they can get involved, of course, is dependent on their strengths and their knowledge and use of body mechanics.

Tennis is a good example. We have many patients who gave up tennis because of their chronically aggravated low back pain. After strengthening their appropriate muscle groups and training them in body mechanics, we accompany them to the tennis court and alter their playing style. The high, hard serve usually requires forced hyperextension of the lumbar spine. By lowering the point at which the ball contacts the racquet, many

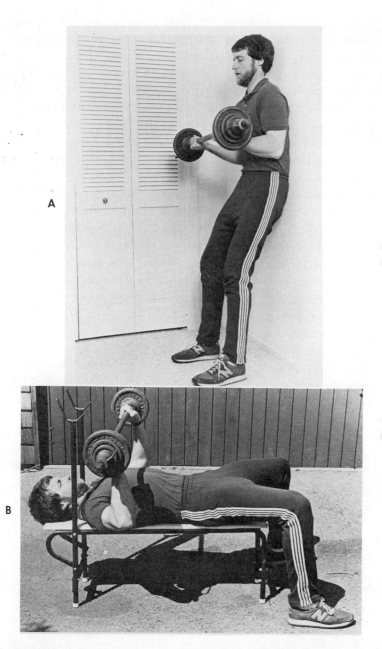

Fig. 8-1. A, Weight lifting against a wall. The wall supports the back. Note the flat back and tightened abdomen.
B, Bench press. Note the flat back.

patients decrease their pain. Scrambling after low and difficult shots causes the lumbar segments to move beyond their tolerated limits, and pain is produced in this group of patients. Thus by decreasing the aggressiveness of a patient's game and playing doubles instead of singles tennis, the game can be enjoyed without painful repercussions.

As with tennis, most other sports can be altered and enjoyed. There are always some sports that are too rigorous for a bad back. Some of these sports cannot be altered because they require maximum efforts with total reflex activity with the body somewhat out of control. These include the contact sports such as football, basketball, and ice hockey. Boxing and wrestling usually have to be avoided. Handball usually requires too much bending and is too fast to allow most people to control their body mechanics. Racquetball is a bit better than the preceding sports except for tennis. Baseball is slow enough except for sliding into bases and the rare fall or collision.

Jogging, of course, can be done except by those with more severe pain. The smoothness of the gait and the speed at which the runner performs are very important. As we speed up, we tend to go into more lumbar lordosis, which is not tolerated in many conditions. A slow jog can be done with pelvic tilt and a flat lumbar spine. Bicycling is very well tolerated by individuals with spinal stenosis, even when it is severe. With the handlebars adjusted, a person with a bad back can lean on them, keeping his back flat with all flexion occurring at the hips. In this way he gets considerable exercise without pain or damage to his back (Fig. 8-2, *A*).

Soccer is another difficult sport. If played casually, it is usually tolerated, but not by individuals with severe pain. Any loss of body control can be dangerous (Fig. 8-3, *B*). Kicking entails a whipping action of the trunk with lordosis of the lumbar spine (Fig. 8-3, *A*). Rugby is in the same category as football. Table tennis is usually well tolerated.

Golf is oddly enough a borderline sport. During the follow-through of the swing of

A   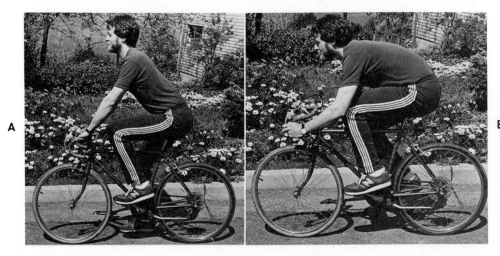   B

Fig. 8-2. Bicycle riding. **A,** Right: back straight and supported by the arms. **B,** Wrong: back bent, bicycle too small, and rider not well supported by the arms.

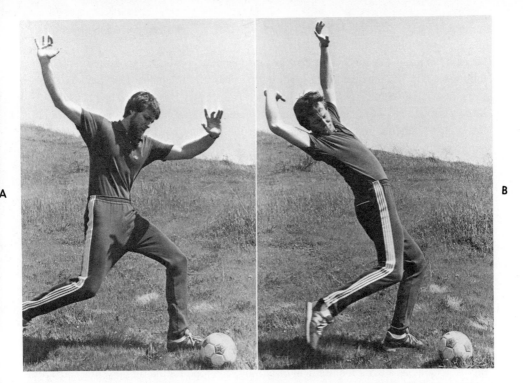

Fig. 8-3. Kicking. **A,** Right: kicker centered over the ball, body balanced, and correct pelvic tilt. **B,** Wrong: kicker off balance and too much lordosis of the spine.

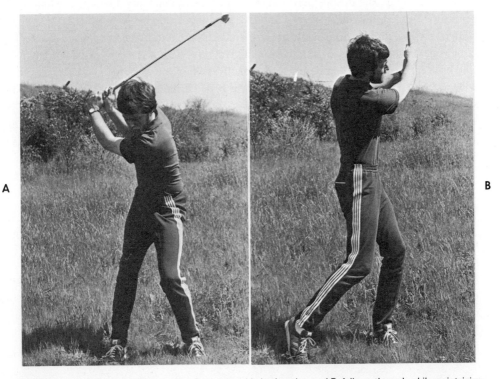

Fig. 8-4. In a correct golf swing the golfer, **A,** shortens his back-swing, and **B,** follows through while maintaining pelvic tilt and keeping stomach tight.

the club, the trunk is poorly controlled by most people. This leaves an injured facet or disc unprotected. If the damaged area is located so that it is traumatized by the swing, then even the patient with the moderately bad back cannot play this sport. The backswing and follow-through can be controlled while a pelvic tilt and straight back are maintained (Fig. 8-4). Some patients find golf almost therapeutic. It may have some relationship to the common form of chiropractic manipulation, which involves twisting the trunk on the pelvis.

ATHLETIC TRAINING PROGRAM

The patients have already learned the basic exercises presented in Chapter 4. They now begin to increase their endurance for performing those basic exercises, to the extent of holding an abdominal sit-up for 5 to 10 minutes and a wall slide for that same amount of time. This amount of endurance and strength allows them to hold their spine in a safe position for long enough periods to accomplish most athletic endeavors. While holding their spine in a safe position with these muscles, they can now go on to develop other muscle groups.

Some patients find it difficult to understand why upper extremity strength is important for protection of the spine. We explain this to them by examples such as the following: A person has a work requirement of pulling on a rope for the riggings of a ship. If the person is generally weak and thin, he has to use all of the effort of his body, including his back. He has to put himself through various contortions to get mechanical advantage. The forces on his spine and the positions can be dangerous. If that individual is a very strong, generally muscled individual, he can almost casually position his spine and do all of the work of pulling with his arms while his legs and abdominal trunk muscles place the trunk in the safest position (Fig. 6-25). This is the way it is with a baseball player or bowler who has very strong upper extremities. He can do much of the work with his arms and not with his spine. Almost all sports are performed better if there is general well-distributed strength and coordination.

To develop this overall general strength and endurance, it takes a fair amount of time and very little specific education and instruction. The safest and most convenient means for us to provide this athletic back school is in conjunction with a sports medicine facility. A sports medicine facility can be a professional gym with special machines for weight lifting, or it can simply be a high school gym with barbells, dumbbells, and a few other pieces of athletic equipment. In a sports medicine facility the trainer is present to demonstrate the use of the equipment in a safe fashion. The back school instructor, however, needs to take the patient through the complete exercise program with regard to his spine before leaving him on his own. The basic instruction for any of this equipment is to first stabilize the spine with the use of the pelvic tilt and abdominal set. If it is at all possible to do the exercises with the back flat on a firm surface, this is the best starting position. Most of the specialized machines for weight lifting, such as the Nautilus and Cybex machines, have seats with slanted backs (Fig. 8-5, *A*). This gives better support for the spine. Special pads and straps are provided to secure the pelvis and spine in a safe position (Fig.

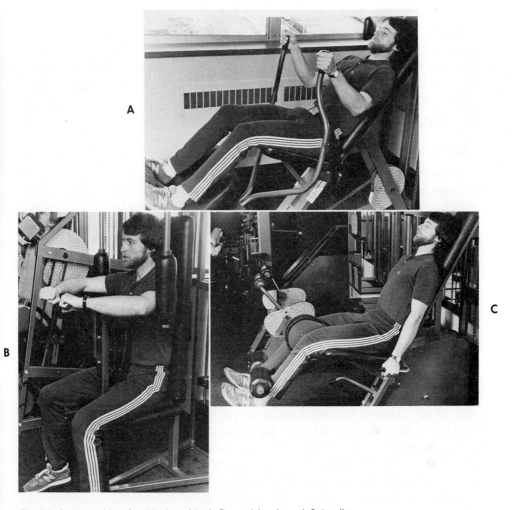

Fig. 8-5. Cybex machine, **A,** with slanted back, **B,** special pads, and, **C,** handles.

8-5, *B*). There are handles on these machines, which further allow stabilizing the trunk while the legs are exercised (Fig. 8-5, *C*).

The basic concepts of athletic training are used. Repetition and tiring of muscles are necessary for maximum development of strength and endurance. Most patients work out 2 or 3 days a week for at least an hour. This continues for 1 or 2 months, until our goals are achieved.

Now that we have developed maximum strength and endurance for this patient's age and condition, we are ready to start the specific training for the athletic endeavor in which he wants to be involved. This requires a back school instructor with a fair knowledge of the sport being taught. If the instructor does not have adequate knowledge, he must go out and study the sport, looking at the body mechanics involved and the effects on the spine. This can be accomplished by participating directly, taking photographs and videotapes, and talking to the patient.

There is not enough space available in this book to dissect every athletic activity to the degree that may be necessary. I take two commonly used sports and examine them. I then go through the athletic activities that can be expected of a patient with moderate and severe pain.

JOGGING AND RUNNING

Jogging is a common "craze" at this time. Probably more patients in my practice are interested in jogging than any other activity. Running is necessary in most sports. Therefore I want to make a relatively thorough study of running and jogging.

If a patient can walk fast, he can jog. Too many joggers with back pain want to return to their previous style of running immediately. This frequently entails too great a stride, too much lumbar lordosis, or too much vertical compression or jarring by having the knee locked in extension at heel strike (Fig. 8-6, *B*). If the individual takes his usual rapid jogging pace and alters the stride by shortening it and bends the knees more throughout the entire running cycle, he will find that there is less jarring (Fig. 8-6, *A*) and a smoother, less traumatic style. This does require more use of the quadriceps muscles to keep the knees bent all of the time. It produces essentially a rapid walk. A patient with back pain can therefore start out walking and then walk faster, until he is doing a smooth jog of this sort. At the same time he should be concentrating on holding a pelvic tilt and keeping his abdominal muscles tightened. This is, of course, totally different and more tiring than his usual jogging method. He has to retrain in this way, starting with 1 or 2 miles and eventually building up to whatever he feels is appropriate. As this style becomes more familiar to him he will find that he is able to maintain the pelvic tilt without great effort and is able to allow his abdominal muscles to relax or reflexly tighten with each step, as occurs with normal jogging. Running is excellent isometric abdominal muscle training.

As the jog becomes a run, the stride is greater, the lumbar curvature is extended, and the jarring is greater. There is a certain amount of this type of trauma that can be allowed with each medical condition of the spine. When it is exceeded, the patient begins having pain and knows that is his limit under his current strength and coordination capabilities.

Other changes can be made in the environment of the athlete who wants to run. The surface on which he runs may make a great deal of difference. Uneven ground with lots of uphill and downhill changes or running on the side of a slope causes the spine to be more greatly taxed. The softness of the surface on which the patient is running and the absorbing quality of the shoes must also be taken into account. Good running shoes offer better stability and distribution of absorption of the vertical jarring forces.

The jogging patient can learn to listen to his feet hitting the ground. When he is doing a fast walk or shuffle, there is little or no sound of his feet hitting the ground. As he becomes more tired or lengthens his stride, he hears his feet hitting the pavement louder and louder. This can be a sign to him that he is tired or should change back to his more protective style. Good warming-up exercises (Fig. 8-7; see also Chapter 4) and lots of

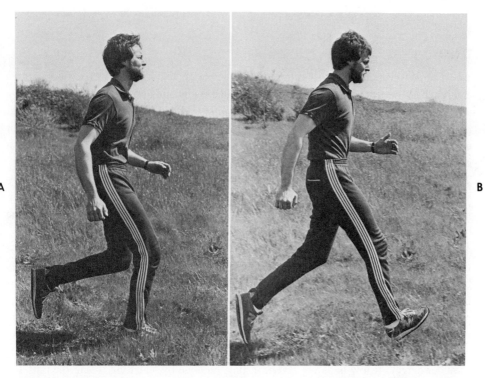

Fig. 8-6. Running. **A,** Right: knee bent, pelvic tilt good, and stride short. **B,** Wrong: knee locked in extension, pelvic tilt poor, and stride too long.

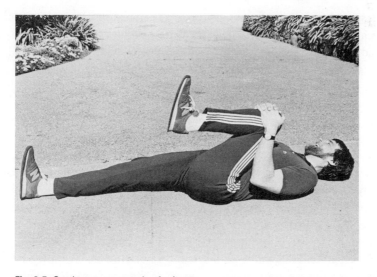

Fig. 8-7. Good warm-up exercise for jogger.

quadriceps work on wall slides or weight lifting further helps strengthen and stabilize the gait for running.

TENNIS

Tennis is a sport that most patients with bad backs can play. It is slow and deliberate enough that a patient can position himself for each swing and does not have to wildly fling around or be out of control of his body mechanics. Playing tennis, especially doubles, provides time for a patient to practice his body mechanics. While standing and waiting for a serve or a ball to be chased, the patient can check his posture to make sure that he is not standing in lordosis. He can practice keeping his knees bent while waiting for a serve. This is the position of activity and readiness for most athletic endeavors that require sudden bursts of activity (Fig. 8-8). Probably the hardest part of playing tennis is reducing the competitive spirit enough that the individual does not feel that he has to go after the hardest hit and the most difficult shots.

When first starting to play after a back injury, the patient can simply hit balls against the backboard. He can then play doubles with a noncompetitive spirit. He can eventually begin to play with people who are not as good at tennis as he is. Eventually as he becomes more sure of himself, he can advance to more competitive opponents. Each time the patient approaches and hits the ball he should be in a good tennis stance with knees bent and abdominal muscles tightened. His backswing and follow-through should not be so much with the trunk as with the arms and shoulders. The ball should generally be hit at shoulder height. If low balls are taken, it must be done by squatting, using the hips and knees rather than bending the lumbar spine. High balls and serves should be allowed to drop before hitting them at such a height that lumbar extension is required (Fig. 8-9).

PROFESSIONAL ATHLETES

Professional athletes and top-flight amateur competitors are a very difficult group with which to deal. They develop small herniated discs or rapid degeneration of discs or facets, and their game can be ruined. They function at 100% efficiency, and this slight pain can take them out of competition. They are already well-developed, have good musculature, and cannot afford to have their body mechanics tampered with very much, if they are going to continue to function at 100% efficiency. We try to make some changes in their game or have them use some form of a brace or support. Sometimes we are able to find an error in their training technique that is setting off their pain. This is particularly true of the swimmer who uses an inner tube to support his feet, while practicing with the upper extremities. This throws him into hyperextension of the lumbar spine and can be a source of pain. Similar errors in rowing by using the back instead of the hips can be the source of back pain. Many changes can be made in the training with regard to warm-up, training techniques, stretching, heat, traction, injections and medications.

Athletes rarely solve their problems simply by reading a back book. Some may benefit if their errors are gross from a group type of program. Even the individualized back school experiences great trouble in returning most athletes to heavy athletics with simple changes in body mechanics and back health care. These individuals are using peak

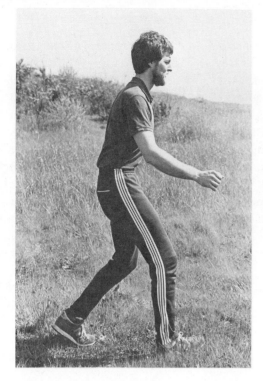

Fig. 8-8. Position of readiness: knees bent, good pelvic tilt, and stomach tight.

A

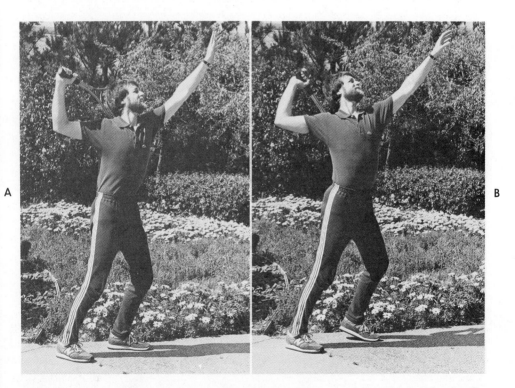

B

Fig. 8-9. Tennis serve. **A,** Right: good pelvic tilt and straight back. The server should wait for the ball to drop. **B,** Wrong: excess lordosis and the reach is too high for the ball.

effort and using their backs heavily. They find it difficult to use substitution motions and still be able to continue to play the sport as they need or want to.

We combined a sports medicine center with a back school. This provides physical therapists and back school instructors who are also athletic trainers. They are very good athletes themselves and are able to develop extreme musculature and train individuals in body mechanics as they would for the Olympics. This requires a special personality on both the part of the patient and the trainer. It frequently requires the ancillary help of injections of cortisone into the facet joints or epidural space, bracing of various sorts, and other training techniques with regard to manipulation, modalities, and equipment changes. With the use of all of our body mechanics knowledge and these tools and techniques, we are able to help most athletes continue the enjoyment of their sport.

9 OTHER CONSERVATIVE MEASURES

Back school lays a foundation for the overall prevention and management of low back pain. There are many other conservative measures that can be added to this foundation. Any one of the other conservative measures might be an even more rapid solution to a particular episode of low back pain. These measures do not, however, carry with them the ability to transfer the responsibility of back care to the patient. They are not going to prevent back pain, give the patient any insight into what caused the pain, and therefore not prevent future episodes. This is one of the major reasons for our current low back pain problem. We return the patient to the same abusive environment and activities from which he came.

Other conservative measures do have value. They are tools that the back school therapists can use at the appropriate time and in specific instances. There are times when the back school therapist should recommend surgery as the most conservative measure to help a patient rapidly return to the most productive life-style possible. The therapist might also recommend or use manipulation, self-mobilization, hanging traction, braces, body jackets, heat, massage, acupuncture, injections, etc.

The following discussion briefly reviews the uses and indications for some of the more popular and, to my way of thinking, more valuable conservative measures.

SELECTION FOR SURGERY

For several decades lumbar surgery has been performed when a patient had progressive neurological deficit and/or continued pain after 2 weeks of bed rest and a positive myelogram. With all of the conservative measures available to us, such a shortsighted view of surgical indications is no longer acceptable. Most, if not all, of the conservative measures presented in this book should be attempted before deciding on a surgical approach.

It is not reasonable to expect a patient with a significant pathological lesion to simply get better by placing him at bed rest. If the patient has a herniated lumbar disc or spinal stenosis with leg pain and slight neurological deficit, little is going to change with bed rest. The pathophysiological lesion is still present. When a patient stands up and begins activity, he is going to produce further nerve root irritation and the pain will return. The bed rest has simply allowed time for the inflammation to subside. It has, in fact, made things worse by weakening the patient so that when he does stand up after 2 weeks, he has much less strength and endurance to use for protective body mechanics. An epidural block or oral cortisone would just as rapidly and completely eliminate the inflammation as the 2 weeks of bed rest.

Something else needs to be done to either change the pathological lesion or the patient's ability to cope. If the pathological lesion is a herniated lumbar disc, the lesion can be altered with various forms of traction, manipulation, injections, and body jackets. The contour of the spine and its curvatures and contents can be altered by posture and exercise training, body jackets, education, and environmental changes. All the back school tools and techniques need to be exhausted before deciding on surgery. Having used all of the back school techniques, if surgery then becomes necessary, its success is more likely. The knowledge and strength obtained during back school is quite likely to prevent the patient from making the same mistakes that he made before surgery. This prevents further pain resulting from instability, late development of degenerative spinal stenosis, and degenerative disc disease at other levels. The surgeon is also better equipped to decide what kind of surgery to perform. The back school helps identify the patient's pain tolerance, strengths, and educational capabilities and in general answers the following question: Does this patient need minor or major surgery?

If this is the first episode of low back pain in a relatively young patient with a verified herniated lumbar disc and no complicating factors, such as spinal stenosis, weakness, or obesity, minor surgery is statistically very successful. Ninety-two percent of these patients improve with a small laminectomy or laminotomy and simple disc excision. They also do well with microsurgery. If a good minor surgery is desirable, the best approach is probably chemonucleolysis in this type of case. Seventy-eight percent of well-selected patients return to normal with an injection of chymopapain, if they have no complications such as spinal stenosis or secondary gain. If there are complicating factors, however, such as long-range recurrent pain from degenerative lumbar disc disease, developing spinal stenosis, weakness, inability to train, learn, and use good body mechanics, low pain tolerances, or secondary gain, the success rate with minor surgery is closer to 50%. These types of patients continue to abuse their backs, develop spinal stenosis at the level of a laminectomy and disc excision, develop further degenerative disc disease at adjacent levels that frequently are already partially deteriorated, and are unable to cope with such pain because of low pain tolerances and poor strength and body mechanics. In such cases it is reasonable to do major surgery, incorporating a fusion at the level operated on primarily and even fusion of other levels, which are quite likely to be the sources of pain in the near future. Discograms and flexion extension films can help identify these potentially painful levels. At the time of surgery direct observation and palpation of these levels and even discograms can be helpful. A one-, two-, or three-level lumbar laminectomy and fusion might be a conservative thing to do in certain groups. We have been doing Knodt rod and Harrington rod fusions in this group of patients who previously had only a 55% success rate. Their success rate now is 78%. Surgeons who have been using posterior interbody fusions for years have found that their success rate is much higher than with a laminectomy alone in these difficult types of cases.

MANIPULATION AND MOBILIZATION

Manipulation is an extremely common and valuable conservative tool. Although there is no good, absolute scientific proof that manipulation works or for what condition it works best, it has been used extensively and successfully in almost every country for centuries. Every day in our spine pain center we see patients who come to us after many years of relief by manipulation. We use and study various forms of mobilization and manipulation. We have developed what seems to work best for our population of patients.

The principle of manipulation or mobilization of the spine seems to be that of placing a particular segment of the spine or several segments through a range of motion slowly or rapidly which results in the reduction of pain, muscle spasm, and improved range of motion. What can such manipulation do? It may be altering the neurophysiology, circulation, soft tissue, or position and alignment of the segments. The position of nucleus pulposus material in fissures and tears of the anulus may be altered by these techniques. Facet joint alignment or synovial imposition in the joint may be changed. The position of nerve roots in the lateral foramina and their association with bone spurs and bulging discs may be altered.

Whatever the reason that manipulation or any other technique works, if it works, its success should be demonstrable to the patient or any impartial observer relatively rapidly and consistently. We should not impose on the patients techniques that are not demonstrably successful. We should not fool ourselves into thinking that a technique works when it is the natural history of the condition to be resolved spontaneously. This is a hard burden of proof to impose on any technique, but the burden applies equally to all of us. We should not perform surgery after surgery on the same patient if we are not having success. We should not use injection repeatedly if we are not having success, and we should not employ manipulation for weeks and months if that is not successful.

I personally feel that a reasonable trial of manipulation for most low back conditions is two or three attempts. If obvious success is achieved, several more manipulations may be warranted. If there is not good success in 2 weeks, there are many other forms of treatment that may be more successful.

Manipulation should never make a person worse. It should be done with a good knowledge of anatomy and a good neurological evaluation before and after manipulation. Slow motions are generally safer than rapid ones. Manipulations can be done to the painful or painless side. Some are done under traction, some under anesthesia. Many are done in a rotational position of the lumbar spine. Some are done with lumbar flexion with manual traction on the coccyx. Regardless of how they are done, if they are successful, patients can and should be taught how to maintain the improvement and prevent recurrence. They should not be made to think that this is some mysterious form of condition and treatment, and they must not become dependent on any one practitioner or technique. We must be looking for ways to make our patients independent and safe.

Self-mobilizations in my opinion are safer than passive manipulations. Self-mobilization techniques are described well by Robin McKenzie in his book and other writings. It is not described here in any detail. Self-mobilization, however, consists of having the patient place his spine through ranges of motion under varying degrees and positions of weight bearing. Pain patterns are observed. Abnormal postures and positions are corrected and altered. Successful pain-relieving positions are repeated many times. Pain-producing positions and postures are avoided.

BRACES AND BODY JACKETS

Some patients with low back pain are unable or unwilling to practice good body mechanics and back health care to control their low back pain. There can be many reasons for this inability or unwillingness. Basic intelligence, language barrier, personality or cultural factors, and many other circumstances can play a part. Some people cannot dance, and some people cannot pole vault. Teaching body mechanics is easier than both of these, but this concept should be understood.

It is my belief that much of the reason for our epidemic of back problems has to do with some basic coordination and habit patterns that are set up early in childhood. They are somewhat culturally related. We all learn a certain method of bending and lifting early in childhood. We develop fixed styles of sitting, walking, and standing. We become habituated to certain forms of exercise or lack of exercise and stretching. These kinds of factors set up our natural body mechanics and give us limits as to the capacity we are going to have as adults for doing such things as dancing, athletics, and bending and lifting properly. Tight hamstrings and habitual lack of the use of hip and knee motion require excessive use of the lumbar spine and ultimately the abuse and breakdown of the lumbar discs.

If we are unable to break these habit patterns and find that a patient is untrainable for any reason, braces and body jackets can be helpful. Just as braces can reshape our teeth, they can have some holding and reshaping capabilities for our spines. Whether or not these new patterns are maintained has yet to be proven.

The theory behind bracing while in a comfortable position has been used for decades. It seems logical to assume that if a patient can find a comfortable position for his spine in bed or standing, we should be able to maintain that position by external supports so that the patient is comfortable at all times.

The principle of finding a comfortable position and maintaining it permeates much of the back school philosophy and the mobilization theories of McKenzie. There is some scientific basis underlying this principle. Anulus tear can be altered in the laboratory by flexion and extension. Intradiscal pressures change with flexion and extension. Clinically, anulus tears seem to improve in an extension position and facet syndromes and certain other disc syndromes seem to improve in a flexion position. From a purely empirical basis the use of the comfortable position has been used by clinicians for years. Patients go to bed and seem to automatically seek their most comfortable positions. Frequently this is the fetal position. Physicians assume that position is the one the patient should maintain while on his feet. They therefore incorporated body jackets with varying amounts of the trunk and even a leg in a position of maximum comfort.

We try to teach patients to maintain the pelvic tilt when standing or in whatever other position is appropriate. If they are unable to learn and maintain this position, we have the urge to force them in some other way. Corsets and body jackets are one method of achieving this goal.

The classic corset has posterior stays molded to the lumbar curvature, which the corset manufacturer seems to deem average or normal. It sometimes has pulls on the side for extra strength. It can be made of canvas for more strength or elastic, which affords more comfort. All of these simply give some support or warning system for the patient to prevent him from bending. He might develop some intraabdominal pressure to help give extra strength and stability to the spine. There are scientific studies that demonstrate corsets to have significant value. In clinical practice they seem to give patients some form of security and perhaps prevent the last degree or so of motion in some patients with instability or impending nerve root irritation. We have many heavy laborers, such as scavengers, in San Francisco, who wear formidable corsets on a regular basis for work. The corsets seem to allow the workers to do labor that they are otherwise unable to do. The basis of this improvement is unknown to me at this time.

In the past body jackets have often been made of plaster of paris. Although these body jackets, casts, and spica casts are rather cumbersome, they are frequently successful in relieving the patient's pain. When removed, at times, the patient remains pain-free. If his pain returns surgeons feel that a fusion is indicated. They do an internal stabilizing procedure on as many as 5 levels of the lumbar spine on the basis of this clinical trial alone. Considerable theory but little proof exists as to why this principle works. It led to the current and rather widespread use of the flexion body jacket.

The improved use of synthetic materials greatly improved the brace and body jacket industry. Plaster casts are relatively easily converted to plastic in a lightweight, removable form. These forms have been used for scoliosis in the Milwaukee and Boston brace for many years. The flexion body jacket for low back pain was recently popularized by Dr. Raney in San Francisco. The Raney flexion body jacket was originally molded to the patient's lower trunk and upper pelvis by making a plaster of paris mold while the patient sat with an abdominal compression device. This was then converted to a plastic material with air holes and Velcro straps. These can now be measured and fitted without a plaster of paris mold.

A flexion body jacket does create a fair amount of pelvic tilt and lumbar flexion. This flexion is shown repeatedly on myelography to reduce the prominence of bulging discs. This is theoretically a result of the tightening of the posterior longitudinal ligament and anulus. The abdominal compression built into the body jacket theoretically increases intraabdominal pressure, which gives support to the spine and possibly even places the spine in some traction. I know from personal experience that the body jacket definitely discourages range of motion of the lumbar spine.

Clinically we find the flexion body jacket useful for many patients with varying disc herniation and ''mechanical'' back pain that we are unable to control with back school and lesser forms of support. Although these jackets work best for patients who cannot or will not learn and use good body mechanics, there are patients with proven herniated lumbar discs who seem to do quite well with their strength and body mechanics but are unable to maintain perfect positioning throughout an entire day of heavy work. They wear these jackets for months and even years. According to Dr. Raney's studies, after a few months the patient should be able to be weaned off the jacket and placed in an exercise program. The alteration of the posture may remain. Most of our patients need the jacket permanently, or at least intermittently, for an indefinite period of time. It is my belief that the flexion body jacket, as with manipulation and hanging traction, can temporarily alter a variety of bulging discs and spinal stenotic syndromes. If the patient, however, returns to his usual abusive activities, the bulge eventually returns or the stenosis redevelops. This, of course, is the natural history of the development of most low back pain. With time, our discs become weaker and lose height, the anulus bulges, the facets override, and the foramina narrow. We can pull them, push them, or cajole them back to nature's original position but the nature of our vertical posture and the needs of people in industrialized societies continue to work against us and the aging process must go on. With the constant vigilance of back school and body mechanics, we can slow down this aging process and reverse it partially and temporarily.

GRAVITY LUMBAR TRACTION

Gravity lumbar traction has been used for centuries to help relieve low back pain. Patients seem to have some natural tendency to feel that they want to be stretched out. This is understandable from a physiological standpoint. The vertical upright posture leads to progressive collapse and shortening of the spine. We are all perhaps trying to keep ourselves stretched out to our original height. From a slightly more scientific but far from proven standpoint, the spinal stenosis and bulging disc phenomenon of the vertical quadriped with lumbar lordosis is at least temporarily reduced with traction and reduction of the lordosis.

Gravity lumbar traction was first brought to my attention in the late 1960s by Victor Steele, who developed a hanging traction device by which the patient hangs upside down over an upper thigh support with his hips flexed at right angles. This seems to reduce the lumbar curvature and is quite comfortable and relieving for me and many of my patients. I used this in my office for several years and prescribed it for patients who still find it valuable. There are many other forms of gravity lumbar traction, including boots, frames, and harnesses. The current most popular form of gravity lumbar traction seems to be that advocated by Charles Burton at the Sister Kenny Institute in Minneapolis, and the gravity guidance system.

MEDICATIONS

Medication is probably the most abused of all conservative measures for low back pain problems. Medication certainly does not place the responsibility of back care on the patient. It feeds into what might be considered a "pill-crazy" society. Antiinflammatory medications do experimentally relieve inflammation. Many back pain conditions have inflammation as a primary causative factor. Muscle relaxants have experimentally been shown to relieve muscle spasm, which plays a part in many low back pain conditions. Analgesics relieve pain, which is the primary subject about which we are speaking. Tension is frequently involved in low back pain conditions, and certain medications seem to reduce emotional tensions. Despite all of the preceding, medications cover up the underlying condition and disguise it. The patient is then less able to monitor his own condition and control it. He becomes more active under the influence of the medication than his condition should allow. The medication wears off, the resultant irritation from the activity gives him more pain, inflammation, or muscle spasm, and he requires more medication. The patient is soon taking more medication and becoming addicted or developing side effects, which then compound and cloud the original condition. When appropriately used as an adjunct to back school, medication can definitely have its place, if its use is well monitored.

INJECTIONS

Many injection techniques are described earlier in the diagnostic sections of this book. Injections can be used strictly therapeutically in the form of trigger-point injections, facet injections, and epidural-cortisone and anesthetic injections. These injections, similar to the previous section on medication, do not transfer the responsibility to the patient. They simply reduce inflammation or stop pain temporarily. This allows the patient to progress more rapidly toward rehabilitation and may shorten the clinical course of his disease. The closer that we can get to the origin of the pain, the more likely it is that the pain is going to be relieved. Taking cortisone by mouth to reduce inflammation in a facet joint can require large amounts, which carries with it complications. Placing a needle in the facet joint carries with it specific complications; it requires less cortisone in a more exact location.

There are tremendous placebo effects with injections. The practitioner must weigh many factors in the decision as to what conservative measure should be applied. Many patients do not like to take medication and most do not like injections. Some people are afraid of manipulations, but most seem to like heat and massage. In my own practice injections are most appropriately used in the more severe cases, when the patient is facing hospitalization or days to weeks of bed rest and other simpler conservative measures fail. Epidural blocks work best for nerve root irritation syndrome from herniated disc, spinal stenosis, or spondylolisthesis. Facet blocks work best for facet arthritis syndrome.

DISCUSSION

Manipulation, braces, and traction have been around for centuries. Their popularity in various forms has waxed and waned. With the development and organization of the spine specialist, we are having a fresh look at these techniques with increasing scientific investigation. I believe that each of these techniques will find its own place in the management of spinal problems. Having devoted my entire career to the investigations and use of every viable spinal technique of which I am aware, the following discussion desribes the place that each of the techniques holds in my spinal practice.

Back pain with an acute onset, as has been stated previously, is at first a self-limiting process. This probably represents anulus tear or perhaps facet injuries that resolve spontaneously. They seem to resolve faster with chiropractic manipulations, McKenzie's mobilization, traction, manipulation, and injections with steroids. The patient should not continue to reinjure the disc or facet joint. The only advantage that back school has over other techniques is that it insists on giving the patient responsibility to stop creating the lesion. Placing the injured part in its most comfortable position, holding it there, and not reinjuring it clears up the condition within a few days. There is less of a tendency for it to recur and become a chronic condition.

Chronic back pain in the form of chronic degenerative disc disease and spinal stenosis only temporarily, if at all, responds to manipulation, mobilization, traction, or injection. It responds best to bracing or back school.

Acute leg pain that is usually a result of a herniated lumbar disc or nerve root irritation from spinal stenosis or spondylolisthesis responds most rapidly to an epidural block and cortisone injection. Occasionally manipulation or mobilization can free an entraped nerve root but just as often it can aggravate the condition. Bracing can at times hold the nerve root in a free position so that it can then recover spontaneously. Back school similarly can teach the person to keep the nerve root in its most comfortable position and not to create the condition again.

There is a variety of chronic back pain that is minor but aggravating in nature. It does not show the gross radiographic changes of chronic degenerative disc disease. It seems to be more related to posture and stiffness than it does to inflammation from recurrent abuse and mechanical reproducible back pain. This pain improves with manipulation, mobilization, and general exercise.

Acupuncture, hypnosis, sclerosing agents, biofeedback, ultrasound, diathermy, pool therapy, shoe lifts, trigger-point injections, diet, and vitamins do not seem to have any consistently greater benefits for one condition over another. All of them are available to us and are used by practitioners in our immediate community.

When a patient comes to our multidisciplinary spinal center, he has all of the conservative measures just listed available to him. The flow and use of these conservative measures is not rigidly controlled but seems to be developed by what works best.

SUMMARY

Other conservative measures superimposed on the foundation of back school have some value in more rapidly returning a patient to normal activity. They all have the danger of making the patient dependent rather than independent. They all have their own specific potential complications and require learning to use the technique to best advantage for the population with whom the therapist is dealing. These other conservative measures should be used for as short a time as possible and should not make the patient any worse or add to the already confusing picture of low back pain.

10 THE FUTURE OF BACK SCHOOL

This is only the beginning. We have already helped 500 other back schools get started around the world. Each of them is taking this basic information and developing it in a form that is specifically valuable to its particular needs and community.

Some back schools have taken on a totally industrial inclination. They align themselves with either the industrial employer, union, vocational rehabilitation consultant, or insurance company that carries the workman's compensation insurance for that industry. The back school instructor learns everything that he can about the particular employees and their jobs. He obtains facilities and equipment in his back school that closely simulate the job of the particular group of employees he is treating. The vocational rehabilitation consultant is primarily interested in returning the patient to a job that he is capable of doing. These consultants serve as an important communications link between the patient, industry, and insurance company. One back school has a vocational rehabilitation consultant as the primary patient manager. The consultant actually escorts the patient to the back school and assures that there is no loss of communication between the involved parties.

There is no end to the degree that specialty back school can be developed. We need to add all forms of sophisticated psychosocial assistance to the basic back school concept. The back school, as we have dealt with it up to this point, involves mostly the physical aspects of the disease and the body mechanics and training to control it. The science of the psychological aspects of industrial injuries and the emotional impact on the patient and society is clearly a most rewarding and necessary area for future development. Fortunately industries, insurance companies, and lawmakers involved with vocational rehabilitation are all becoming aware of and lending their financial support to this type of development. We are currently devising a well-controlled research project to verify the benefit of back school in industry. Statistically we have already found great monetary savings and decreases in back injuries in the Southern Pacific Transportation Companies and Safeway Stores, Inc. Further research is necessary to find better means of prevention at the industrial level.

One of the most exciting and yet untouched areas of the future of back school is in schools themselves. At what age do the bad back health care habits and bad body mechanics that lead to back injuries develop (Fig. 10-1)? Is there some physical makeup of a child that leads him into bad habits toward back health care? Can these patterns be identified? At what age can a child be taught to change his body mechanics and back

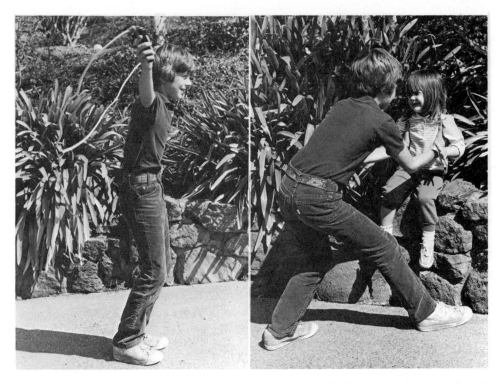

Fig. 10-1. At what age can a child be taught good back health care habits and good body mechanics?

health care habits? Will changing the seating arrangements in schools lead to better backs for our youth?

Scoliosis screening programs are very successful in identifying scoliosis early and treating it before it reaches a stage of severe curvature and disability. School nurses who are screening for scoliosis could similarly be trained to look at the back health care habits, lifting techniques, and body mechanics of our children. Perhaps early identification of bad body mechanics habits could be identified and eliminated with early remedial training. This could and should be taught in health classes and health education in high schools and colleges.

Another area of potential back injury and poor back health habits is in the athletic areas of our schools. Are some of the exercises we have been teaching our children for years detrimental to their spines? We certainly find in the adult that the exercise programs that we did in high school frequently precipitate and usually aggravate the degenerative spines of the middle-aged patients.

Intraabdominal pressure monitoring seems to have some great research possibilities. There are certain patterns of use of the abdominal musculature, which creates increased intraabdominal pressure at the appropriate time for various lifting tasks. As these patterns and techniques are discovered and taught in back schools, we will evolve new teaching techniques. A patient could swallow a pressure pill and then observe his abdominal pressure development during a given task and compare it with that which has been found to be most efficient and protective.

Manipulation and traction have been successful for centuries in relieving back pain. We have never identified exactly the reason they are successful or on which patients they are most successful. There are no good, double-blind, well-controlled studies on these areas. Back schools need to continue evaluating these techniques and trying to verify when they should be used. Eventually we will be able to teach patients to manipulate or put traction on their own spines at home to correct postural problems, reduce intradiscal pressure, change the alignment of an acutely painful spine, and control chronic low back pain.

Nutrition has been virtually untouched in the back school area. We do not know what information to give our patients to help them keep good nourishment in the vertebral segments. Dr. Nachemson demonstrated that vertical loading, as in jogging, seems to give better nourishment to the discs. What are the exercises that best supply blood and nutrients to the discs? What foods might be valuable and what foods or environmental exposures may be detrimental?

The psychology of low back pain and pain in general is a burgeoning field. Pain clinics are sprouting up all over the country. Back schools are frequently associated with pain clinics or at least a psychologist or pain control specialist. Transcutaneous stimulators, hypnosis, biofeedback, and acupuncture are all being used for pain control. What are the physical and psychological effects of these modalities? We again have no well-controlled studies to verify what they are actually doing or whether they are any better than the natural healing process or other techniques discussed in this book. When does pain behavior become more significant than the physical condition? Are there faster and easier methods of altering pain behavior than the currently used behavioral modification techniques? Can we identify some of the pain patterns early in childhood and begin altering them before they become so deeply ingrained that the patient seeks surgery after surgery for an essentially psychological process? Can the areas of self-analysis, self-actualizations, enlightenment training, etc. be used to help change a patient's attitude toward his body and his pain? How can these psychological movements be incorporated in standard psychotherapy to treat larger numbers of pain patients, perhaps in groups?

What about yoga, acupressure, osteopuncture, and other pressure and stretching techniques? Do they have a place in back school? We do not know. We pointed out the areas where stretching is known to be of some value. Overstretching of the anulus and facet joints seems to be detrimental, if an individual ascribes to the scientific studies done on rotational strains and damage to the vertebral segment. Certainly keeping structures stretched to a normal degree can be assumed to be helpful or preventive. Invasive techniques of sclerosing agents and needles need considerable research before being widely used. Pain is controlled by many activities of pressure and stretching. As long as these activities do not make the patient dependent, do not become excessively expensive, or do not do any damage, they seem acceptable for pain control. As far as their doing anything that permanently alters the underlying condition, there is no scientific acceptance or verification.

Public education can do for low back pain what has been done for dental hygiene. Much low back pain is preventable and controllable with simple measures that can be reinforced through public education. Most back schools are involved in some way with public education in their hospitals and local communities. Some are producing videotapes and interesting slide and television programs for the public. These require great ingenuity and educational capabilities to be interesting and yet accurate enough to supply the message. Presentation of back health care information in an interesting and valuable fashion is a great challenge. We have made hundreds of attempts at newer and exciting ways of presenting this information. Our best effort to date is presented in a back school package titled *The Back School* and is published by The C.V. Mosby Company. It is presented in a four-part audiovisual program that has a story form with a main character, Dan, who goes through a back school education and training program. He learns his exercises and back school information and becomes somewhat of a convert who carries the information to his family and fellow employees. Other back schools have used comic characters, pantomime, and strictly scientific presentations with stick figure drawings. The challenge is there. The information should be accepted to others by innovative, helpful, and scientific means. The future of back school is now in your hands. The way that you use this information can change the world. The current epidemic of back pain is preventable and controllable.

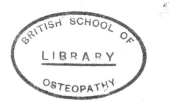

REFERENCES AND SUGGESTED READINGS

American Academy of Orthopaedic Surgeons: Symposium on the lumbar spine, St. Louis, 1981, The C.V. Mosby Co.

American Academy of Orthopaedic Surgeons: Symposium on the spine, St. Louis, 1967, The C.V. Mosby Co.

Andersson, G., Örtengren, R., and Nachemson, A.: Quantitative studies of back loads in lifting, Spine 1:178-185, 1976.

Andersson, G., Örtengren, R., and Nachemson, A.: Intradiskal pressure intra-abdominal pressure and myoelectric back muscle activity related to posture and loading, Clin. Orthop. 129:156-164, 1977.

Andersson, G., Örtengren, R., and Nachemson, A.: Quantitative studies of the load on the back in different working postures, Scand. J. Rehabil. Med. (suppl.) 6:173-181, 1978.

Andersson, G., Örtengren, R., and Nachemson, A.: Studies of back loads in fixed spinal postures and in lifting, Safety in manual materials handling, Washington, D.C., 1979, U.S. Department of Health, Education and Welfare, pp. 26-33.

Andersson, B.J.G., et al.: Lumbar disc pressure and myoelectric back muscle activity during sitting. I. Studies on an experimental chair, Scand. J. Rehabil. Med. 6:104-114, 1974.

Andersson, G., and Schultz, A.B.: Effects of fluid injections on mechanical properties of intervertebral discs, J. Biomech. 12:453-458, 1979.

Armstrong, J.R.: Lumbar disc lesions, London, 1976, E.S. Livingstone.

Asmussen, E.: The weight carrying function of the human spine, Acta Orthop. Scand. 29:276, 1960.

Ayoub, M.M.: Human factors, 1973, pp. 265-268.

Ayoub, M.M., Dryden, R.D., and Knipfer, R.E.: Psychophysical based models for the prediction of lifting capacity of the industrial worker Feb. 1976, Society of Automotive Engineers, Inc.

Bartelink, D.L.: The role of abdominal pressure in relieving the pressure on the lumbar intervertebral discs, J. Bone Joint Surg. 39B:718-725, 1957.

Bergquist-Ullman, M., and Larsson, U.: Acute low back pain in industry. A controlled prospective study with special reference to therapy and confounding factors, Acta Orthop. Scand. (suppl.) 170, 1977.

Berkson, M.H., Nachemson, A., and Schultz, A.B.: Mechanical properties of human lumbar spine motion segments. Part II. Responses in compression and shear; influence of gross morphology, J. Biomech. Eng. 101:53-57, 1979.

Bourdillon, J.F.: Spinal manipulation, ed. 2, New York, 1973, Appleton-Century-Crofts.

Brown, J.R.: Manual lifting and related fields, Ottawa, 1976, Ontario Ministry of Labour.

Buerger, A.: Approaches to the validation of manipulation therapy, Springfield, Ill., 1977, Charles C Thomas, Publisher.

Cailliet, R.: Low back pain, Philadelphia, 1964, F.A. Davis Co.

Cailliet, R.: Neck and arm pain, Philadelphia, 1964, F.A. Davis Co.

Cailliet, R.: Scoliosis, diagnosis and management, Philadelphia, 1975, F.A. Davis Co.

Cailliet, R.: Soft tissue pain and disability, Philadelphia, 1978, F.A. Davis Co.

Chaffin, D.B.: Human strength capability and low-back pain, J. Occup. Med. 16:248-254, 1974.

Chaffin, D.B.: Ergonomics guide for the assessment of human static strength, Am. Ind. Hyg. Assoc. J. 36(7):505-511, 1975.

Coyer, A.B., and Curwen, I.H.M.: Low back pain treated by manipulation. A controlled series, Br. Med. J. 1:705-707, 1955.

Cyriax, J.: Textbook of orthopaedic medicine, Vol. 1, Diagnosis of soft tissue lesions, Baltimore, 1975, The Williams & Wilkins Co.

Cyriax, J.: Textbook of orthopaedic medicine, Vol. 2, Treatment by manipulation, massage and injection, Baltimore, 1975, The Williams & Wilkins Co.

Davis, P.R.: Posture of the trunk during the lifting of weights, Br. Med. J. 87-89, Jan. 10, 1959.

Davis, P.R.: The mechanics and movements of the back in working situations, text of lecture, 1966, C.S.P. Annual Congress.

Davis, P.R., Troup, J.D.G., and Burnard, J.H.: Movements of the thoracic and lumbar spine when lifting: a chrono-cyclophotographic study, J. Anat. **99:**13-26, 1975.

Dilke, T.F.W., Burry, H.C., and Grahame, R.: Extradural corticosteroid injection in management of lumbar nerve root compression, Br. Med. J. **2:**635-637, June 1973.

Egbert, L.D., et al.: Reduction of postoperative pain by encouragement and instruction of patients, N. Engl. J. Med. **270:**825-827, 1964.

Fahrni, W.H.: Backache and primal posture, Vancouver, 1976, Musqueam Publishers, Ltd.

Fahrni, W.H.: Backache: assessment and treatment, Vancouver, 1976, Musqueam Publishers, Ltd.

Farfan, H.F.: Mechanical disorders of the low back, Philadelphia, 1973, Lea & Febiger.

Farfan, H.F., editor: Symposium on the lumbar spine, Ortho. Clin. North Am., Vol. 6, No. 1, Philadelphia, Jan. 1975, W.B. Saunders Co.

Fielding, J.W., and Rothman, R.H., editors: Symposium on the lumbar spine II, Orthop. Clin. North Am., Vol. 8, No. 1, Philadelphia, Jan. 1977, W.B. Saunders Co.

Finneson, B.E.: Low back pain, Philadelphia, 1973, J.B. Lippincott Co.

Fisk, J.W.: The painful neck and back, Springfield, Ill. 1977, Charles C Thomas, Publisher.

Floyd, W.F., and Silver, P.H.S.: The function of the erectores spinae muscles in certain movements and postures in man, J. Physiol. **129:**184-203, 1955.

Frankel, V.H., and Burstein, A.H.: Orthopaedic biomechanics, Philadelphia, 1971, Lea & Febiger.

Frankel, V., and Nordin, M., editors: Basic biomechanics of the skeletal system, Philadelphia, 1980, Lea & Febiger.

Freeman, M.A.R.: The pathogenesis of primary osteoarthrosis: an hypothesis. In Apley, A.G., editor: Modern trends in orthopaedics, Vol. 6, Kent, England, 1972, Butterworth & Co. (Publishers) Ltd., pp. 40-94.

Glover, J.R., Morris, J.G., and Khosla, T.: Back pain: a randomized clinical trial of rotational manipulation of the trunk, Br. J. Ind. Med. **31:**59-64, 1974.

Hall, H.: Paper presented at a meeting of the International Society for the Study of the Lumbar Spine, San Francisco, 1978.

Hanman, B.: The evaluation of physical ability, N. Engl. J. Med. **258(20):**986-993, 1958.

Healy, K.M.: Does preoperative instruction make a difference? Am. J. Nurs. **68:**62, Jan. 1968.

Helfelt, A.J., and Gruebel, D.M.: Disorders of the lumbar spine, Philadelphia, 1978, J.B. Lippincott Co.

Hoppenfeld, S.: Physical examination of the spine and extremities, New York, 1976, Appleton-Century-Crofts.

Hoppenfeld, S.: Orthopaedic neurology, Philadelphia, 1977, J.B. Lippincott Co.

Horst, M., and Brinckmann, P.: Measurement of stress distribution on the endplate of the vertebral body. Volvo Awards Prize, 1980. Spine **6:**217, 1981.

Jayson, M.: The lumbar spine and back pain, New York, 1976, Grune & Stratton, Inc.

Jorgensen, K.: Back muscle strength and body weight as limiting factors for work in the standing slightly-stooped position, Scand. J. Rehabil. Med. **2:**149-153, 1970.

Kane, R.L., et al.: Manipulating the patient. A comparison of the effectiveness of physician and chiropractor care, Lancet **1:**1333-1336, 1974.

Kaye, R.L., and Hammond, A.H.: Understanding rheumatoid arthritis. Evaluation of a patient education program, J.A.M.A. **239(23):**2466-2467, 1978.

Kendall, P.H., and Jenkins, J.M.: Exercises for backache: a double-blind controlled trial, Physiotherapy **54:**154-157, 1968.

Klausen, K.: The form and function of the loaded human spine, Acta Physiol. Scand. **65:**176-190, Sept.-Oct. 1965.

Klausen, K., and Asmussen, E.: Form and function of the erect human spine, Clin. Orthop. **25:**55, 1962.

LaRocca, H., and Macnab, I.: Value of pre-employment radiographic assessment of the lumbar spine, Can. Med. Assoc. J. **101:**383-388, 1969.

Levine, P.H., and Britten, A.F.: Supervised patient-management of hemophilia. A study of 45 patients with hemophilia A and B, Ann. Intern. Med. **78:**195-201, 1973.

Lidström, A., and Zachrisson, M.: Physical therapy on low back pain and sciatica. An attempt at evaluation, Scand. J. Rehabil. Med. **2:**37-42, 1970.

McKenzie, R.A.: The lumbar spine, mechanical diagnosis and therapy 1981, Spinal Publications.

Macnab, I.: Backache, Baltimore, 1977, The Williams & Wilkins Co.

Magora, A.: Investigation of the relation between low back pain and occupation, Industr. Med. Surg. **39**:465-471, 1970.

Magora, A.: Investigation of the relation between low back pain and occupation. V. Psychological aspects, Scand. J. Rehabil. Med. **5**:191-196, 1973.

Magora, A., and Taustein, I.: An investigation of the problem of sick-leave in the patient suffering from low back pain, Indstr. Med. Surg. **38**:398-408, 1969.

Maigne, R.: Orthopedic medicine, Springfield, Ill. 1976, Charles C Thomas, Publisher.

Maitland, G.D.: Vertebral manipulation ed. 4, Woburn, Mass., 1977, Butterworth (Publishers) Inc.

Mennel, J.: Back pain, Boston, 1960, Little, Brown & Co.

Mennel, J.: Joint pain, Boston, 1960, Little, Brown & Co.

Miller, L.V., and Goldstein, J.: More efficient care of diabetic patients in a county-hospital setting, N. Engl. J. Med. **286**:1388-1391, 1972.

Mooney, V.: Alternative approaches for the patient beyond the help of surgery, Orthop. Clin. North Am. **6**:331-334, 1975.

Morris, J.M., Lucas, D.B., and Bresler, B.: Role of the trunk in stability of the spine, J. Bone Joint Surg. **43-A**:327-351, 1961.

Nachemson, A.: Measurement of intradiscal pressure. Acta Orthop. Scand. **28**:269-289, 1959.

Nachemson, A.: Lumbar intradiscal pressure. Acta Orthop. Scand. (suppl.) **43**:1-104, 1960.

Nachemson, A.: Some mechanical properties of the lumbar intervertebral discs, Bull. Hosp. Joint. Dis. (New York) **23**:130-143, 1962.

Nachemson, A.: The influence of spinal movements on the lumbar intradiscal pressure and on the tensile stresses in the anulus fibrosus. Acta Orthop. Scand. **33**:183-207, 1963.

Nachemson, A.: The effect of forward leaning on lumbar intradiscal pressure. Acta Orthop. Scand. **35**:314-328, 1965.

Nachemson, A.: Physiotherapy for low back pain patients. A critical look, Scand. J. Rehabil. Med. **1**:85-90, 196.

Nachemson, A.: Towards a better understanding of low back pain. A review of the mechanics of the lumbar disc, Rheumatol. Rehabil. **14**:129-143, 1975.

Nachemson, A.: Lumbar intradiscal pressure. In Jayson, M., editor: The lumbar spine and back pain, New York, 1976, Grune & Stratton, Inc., pp. 257-269.

Nachemson, A.: The lumbar spine. An orthopaedic challenge, Spine **1**:59-71, 1976.

Nachemson, A., and Elfström, G.: Intravital dynamic pressure measurements in lumbar discs. A study of common movements, maneuvres and exercises, Scand. J. Rehabil. Med. (suppl.) **1**:1-40, 1970.

Nachemson, A., and Evans, J.: Some mechanical properties of the third human lumbar interlaminar ligament (ligamentum flavum), J. Biomech. **1**:211-220, 1968.

Nachemson, A., and Lindh, M.: Measurement of abdominal and back muscle strength with and without low back pain, Scand. J. Rehabil. Med. **1**:60-63, 1969.

Nachemson, A., and Morris, J.: In vivo measurements of intradiscal pressure, J. Bone Joint. Surg. **46A**:1077-1092, 1964.

Nachemson, A., Schultz, A.B., and Berkson, M.H.: Mechanical properties of human lumbar spine motion segments. Influences of age, sex, disc level and degeneration, Spine **4**:1-8, 1979.

Örtengren, R., et al.: Vocational electromyography: studies of localized muscle fatigue at the assembly line, Ergonomics **18**:157-174, 1975.

Örtengren, R., Lindström, L., and Petersén, I.: Periodic muscle loading. Objective quantification and prediction of muscle fatigue [In Swedish], Project report to the Swedish Work Environment Fund, Göteborg, 1978, University of Göteborg, Department of Clinical Neurophysiology.

Park, K.S., and Chaffin, D.B.: Prediction of maximum loads for manual materials handling, Professional Safety, May 1975.

Patient Care Editors: Back and neck pain, 1977, Wallace Laboratories.

Payton, O.D., Hirt, S., and Newton, R.A.: Neurophysiologic approaches to therapeutic exercise, Philadelphia, 1977, F.A. Davis Co.

Pedersen, O.F., Petersen, R., and Staffeldt, E.S.: Back pain and isometric back muscle strength of workers in a Danish factory, Scand. J. Rehabil. Med. Vol. 7, 1975.

Pre-employment strength testing, Pub. No. 77-163, May 1977, NIOSH Technical Information.

Roozbazar, A.: Biomechanics of lifting. In Nelson, R.C., and Morehouse, C.A., editors: Biomechanics IV, Balitmore, 1974, University Park Press, pp. 19-29.

Rothman, R., and Simeone, F.: The Spine, Vol. 1 and 2, Philadelphia, 1975, W.B. Saunders Co.

Rowe, M.L.: Low back pain in industry. A position paper, J. Occup. Med. **11:**161-169, 1969.

Shephard, R.J., and Lavallee, H.: Physical fitness assessment: principles, practice, and application, Springfield, Ill., 1978, Charles C Thomas, Publisher.

Snook, S.H.: Low back pain in industry, Asse Journal, April 1972.

Snook, S.H., and Ciriello, V.M.: Maximum weights and work loads acceptable to female workers, J. Med. **16:**527-534, 1974.

Stolley, P.D., and Kuller, H.H.: The need for epidemiologists and surgeons to cooperate in the evaluation of surgical therapies, Surgery **78:**123-125, 1975.

Stubbs, D.A.: Trunk stresses in construction and other industrial workers, Spine **6:**83, 1981.

Tichauer, E.R.: Occupational biomechanics, 1975, Institute of Rehabilitation Medicine, New York University Medical Center.

Troup, J.D.G.: The biomechanics of the spine, Spinal Orthotic

Troup, J.D.G., and Chapman, A.E.: The static strength of the lumbar erectores spinae, J. Anat. **105:**186, 1969.

Vasey, J.R., and Crozier, L.W.: Basic movement patterns and their relationship to occupational physical problems, Glasgow, April 1977, Royal Infirmary, School of Physiotherapy.

Wernstein, P., et al.: Lumbar spondylosis, Chicago, 1977, Year Book Medical Publishers, Inc.

Westrin, C-G.: Low back sick-listing. A nosological and medical insurance investigation, Scand. J. Soc. Med. (suppl.) **7:**1-116, 1973.

White, A.A., and Panjabi, M.M.: Clinical biomechanics of the spine, Philadelphia, 1978, J.B. Lippincott Co.

White, A.H.: Evaluation of the chronic pain patient. In American Academy of Orthopaedic Surgeons: Symposium on the lumbar spine, St. Louis, 1981, The C.V. Mosby Co.

White, A.H.: Low back patient goes to school. In American Academy of Orthopaedic Surgeons: Symposium on the lumbar spine, St. Louis, 1981, The C.V. Mosby Co.

White, A.H.: Optimistic reoperation for chronic lumbar spine pain. In American Academy of Orthopaedic Surgeons: Symposium on the lumbar spine, St. Louis, 1981, The C.V. Mosby Co.

White, A.H., et al.: The back school: an audiovisual team approach to low back pain, St. Louis, 1981, The C.V. Mosby Co.

White, A.W.M.: Low back pain in men receiving workmen's compensation: a follow-up study. Can. Med. Assoc. J. **101:**61-67, 1969.

Wilkinson, M.: Cervical spondylosis, its early diagnosis and treatment, Ottawa 1976, Ontario Ministry of Labour.

Williams, P.C.: Low back and neck pain, Springfield, Ill., 1976, Charles C Thomas, Publisher.

Wiltse, L., and Ruge, D.: Spinal disorders, diagnosis and treatment, Philadelphia, 1977, Lea & Febiger.

Zachrisson, M.: The low back pain school, Danderyd, Sweden, 1972, Danderyd's Hospital.

Zohn, D.A., and Mennel, J.M.: Diagnosis and physical treatment of musculoskeletal pain, Boston, 1976, Little, Brown & Co.

INDEX

A

Abdominal compression, 72
Activities
  daily, 118-134
  household, 120-123
    ergonomics of, 134-136
Acupuncture, 176
Analgesics, 174
Anesthetics, spinal, diagnostic, 23-24
  potential complications with, 24
Ankylosing spondylitis, 28-29t, 36
Anulus tear, 27, 28-29t, *30*, 84
Arthritis, facet, 28-29t, 35
Arthrogram, facet, 25
Athletes, professional, 166-168
Athletic training program, 162-164; *see also* Back school, athletic
Athletics, 147-168

B

Back injuries
  investigation of, 145
  management of, 144-146
  prevention of, 143-144
Back pain; *see* Pain, back; *see also* Low back pain
Back school
  athletic, 147-168
  basic, 48-81
    day one, 49-67
    day two, 68-76
    day three, 76-77
    day four, 78
    examination, before and after, *68-69*
    exercises, 74
    general obstacle course testing, 53-64
    goals and schedules, 50, 70-71, 77, 78
    obstacle course, 49-52
    patient instruction, 72-74
    variations on, 79

Back school—cont'd
  basic—cont'd
    working patient in, 74-76
  development of concept of, 44-45
  future of, 177-180
  history of, 43-47
  in the home environment, 107-140
    and bed rest, 107-112
    and daily activities, 118-134
    ergonomics of, 134-138
    and patient evaluation, 139-140
    and sitting, 112-117
    and standing and walking, 117
  hospital, 82-106
    before and after surgical hospital program, 93-94
    extended day care program in, 95-96
    inpatient acute conservative care program in, 84-93
    pain rehabilitation inpatient program in, 94-95
    and program flow, 83
  industrial, 79; *see also* Back school in the work environment
  remedial, 47, 145
  statistics, 45-47
  in the work environment, 141-156
    dilemma of, 141-143
    solution for, 143-146
    work task and environment design in, 146-156
Backbend, straight, *58*
Barca lounger, 116
Bathing, 137-138
Bed
  Circ-O-Lectric, 84
  getting out of, 112
  making, 133
  Nelson, 84, 90, 93
  water, 107
Bed exercise routine, progressive, 88t
Bed rest, 107-112
Bedding, 107

Italicized numbers indicate illustrations.
Material in tables indicated by t.

Behavioral modification, 79, 80, 81, 95
Bending, lateral, 151
Biofeedback, 80, 84, 176
Blocks
 diagnostic, 16
 epidural, 17, 82, 175
  indwelling, 18-22
 facet, 17, 24-25, 175
 selective nerve root, 23
 spinal, diagnostic, 23-24
Blue Cross Association, 45
Body dimensions, standing worker's, 154
Body mechanics, 114, 139
 of bending, 72-74, *73*
Bone scan, 16
Braces and body jackets, 172-174
Bracing after surgery, 93
Bupivacaine, 22
Burton, Charles, 174

C

Care, home self-, 118-120
Carpentry, 129
Carrying
 in home environment, 126-127
 in industry, 150
Catheter, epidural, 18
Chaffin, Donald, 150
Chair(s)
 Ergon, 116
 human, 74, *75*, 127
 types of, 116
 vertebra, 116
 work, 153-154
Chloroprocaine, 21
Chronic degenerative lumbar disc disease, 27,
  28-29t, *31, 32*
Chronic degenerative lumbar segment, 32
Chymopapain, 170
Circ-O-Lectric bed, 84
Climbing and reaching, 132
Clinic, industrial, 145
Clothes, 136
Communication, 142, 145
Complications, potential
 of diagnostic spinal anesthetics, 24
 of indwelling epidural block, 22
Compression
 abdominal, 72
 neurological, 2
Computed tomography scan, 16-17

Conditioning program, operant, 81
Conservative treatment, 169-176
Consultant
 rehabilitation, 140
 vocational, 140
Contour position, 84, *85*
Controls, sitting and standing positions for, 154
Corsets, 91
Cortisone, 89, 168
Crossed straight leg raising, 49
CT scan; *see* Computed tomography scan
Cybex machine, *163*

D

Daily activities, 118-134
Deconditioning process, 142
Degenerating intervertebral segment, 1
Degenerating lumbar segment, 1, 32
Degenerative disc disease, 2, 27, 28-29t, *31,*
  32
Derangement, 26
Design, work task and environment, 146-156
Diagnosis(es)
 fourteen, 26
 potential athletic capabilities by, 157t
 shortcuts to classification in, 39-42
Diathermy, 176
Diet, 176
Disability; *see* Symptoms, athletics and sever-
  ity of
Disc disease, chronic degenerative, 27, 28-29t,
  31, 32
Disc injuries, acute, 84, 87; *see also* Herni-
  ated nucleus pulposus
Discogram, 16, 17, 24, 170
Disease
 chronic degenerative lumbar disc, 27, 28-
  29t, *31, 32*
 degenerative disc, 2
Driving, truck, 155
 reducing low back stress in, 155-156
Dynamic physical evaluation, 14-15
Dysfunction, 26

E

Education
 public, 180
 of the worker, 142, 144
Electromyogram, 16
EMG; *see* Electromyogram
Emotional and social factors, 150

Employees, ongoing reinforcement for, 144
Environment
  design, work task and, 146-156
  home; *see* Back school in the home environment
  kitchen, analysis of, 135
  psychological, 80-81
  work; *see* Back school in the work environment
Environmental considerations, 149-150
Epidural block; *see* Blocks, epidural
Epidural catheter, 18
Epidural venogram, 16, 17
Ergon chair, 116
Ergonomics
  in home environment, 134-138
  in industry, 79; *see also* Design, work task and environment
Etiology, 1-2
Evaluation
  of patient, 1-25
  in home environment, 139-140
  physical
    dynamic, 14-15
    low back test diagnosis, *51; see also* Examination, physical
Examination
  basic back school before and after, *68-69*
  dynamic evaluation, 84
  Pentothal, 24
  physical, 15-16; *see also* Evaluation, physical
Exercise(s)
  basic back school, 74
  during bed rest, 109-111
  encouraging, in truck drivers, 156
  hanging, 158
  knee-to-chest, *90*
  progressive bed, 88t
  stretching, 117
Exercise tolerance test, 76
Extended day care hospital program, 95-96

F

Facet arthritis, 28-29t, 35
Facet arthrogram, 25
Facet block, 17, 24-25, 175
Facet joints, 2
Facet syndrome, 17, 175
Fahrni, Dr. Harry, 44
Fibrosis, intraneural, 34

Flexion extension films, 170
Fluoroscopy, biplane, 24
Fractures, 84, 87
Functional rating scale, 5-6

G

Gardening, 128-129
Goals, basic back school, 50, 70-71, 77, 78
Golf, 160, *161,* 162
Gravitonics gym, 158

H

Hall, Dr. Hamilton, 44
Hamstring stretch, 110
Heat, local, 84
Heat stress, 149
Hendler 10-Minute Screening Test For Chronic Back Pain Patients, 7-9
Herniated nucleus pulposus
  lumbar, 34, 84
  and nerve involvement, 28-29t
  with nerve root irritation, 34
  and neurological deficit, 32, *33,* 34, 87
Hip flexion, 114, 118
History
  of back school, 43-47
  pain, 4
  patient, 2-5
HLAW 27 antigen, 36
Home environment; *see* Back school in the home environment
Home self-care, 118-120
Hospital back school; *see* Back school, hospital
Hospital programs, 96-97
Household activities; *see* Activities, household
Human chair, 74, *75,* 127
Hypnosis, 80, 176

I

Iatrogenic diagnosis, 28-29t, 37
Ice massage, 84
Image intensification, 24
Industrial back injury dilemma, 141
Industrial clinic, 145
Industrial evaluation program, 95
Industry, disinterest in, 143
Injections, 175
  trigger-point, 176

Injuries
  back
    investigation of, 145
    management of, 144-146
    prevention of, 143-144
  extension, 39
  flexion, 39
  industrial, dilemma of, 141-143
Inpatient acute conservative care program,
    84-93
Instruction, patient, basic back school, 66,
    72-74
Intervertebral segment, degenerating, 1, 32
Intraabdominal pressure, 150
  monitoring, 178
Intraneural fibrosis, 34

J

Jackets, braces and body, 172-174
  and flexion, 91, 173
Jogging, 160, 164-166

K

Kitchen environment, analysis of, 135
Knee-chest positions, 15
Knee-to-chest exercise, *90*
Kneeling, 128-129, 133

L

Laboratory studies, 16
Lawn mower, pushing, 129
Leg
  sensory loss in, 49
  weakness of, 49
Leg pain, 40; *see also* Pain, back and leg
  acute, 176
Lidocaine, 20
Lifting
  high frequency of, 148, 149
  in home, 124
  in industry, 147-149
Low back pain; *see also* Pain, back
  acute, 109
  chronic, 40t, 109
  classification of, 26-42
  diagnosis of, shortcuts to, 39-42
  etiology of, and patient evaluation, 1-25
  findings in, and recommended therapy, 28-
    29t
  functional, 38-39
  minor, 42

Low back pain—cont'd
  psychological, 38-39
  psychology of, 179
  therapy for, recommended, findings and,
    28-29t
Lumbago, 26
Lumbar segment, degenerating, 1
Lying position, proper, 107

M

Management of back injuries, 144-146
Manipulation, 179
  and mobilization, 170-171
Marcaine; *see* Bupivacaine
Massage, 84
Mattresses
  "holey," 87
  soft, 107; *see also* Water beds
McKenzie, Robin, 14-15, 171
McKenzie "press-up," *111*
Medications, 174-175
Minnesota Multiphasic Personality Inventory, 5
MMPI; *see* Minnesota Multiphasic Personality
    Inventory
Mobilization, 84
  manipulation and, 170-171
Muscle effort, minimizing, in truck drivers,
    155
Muscle relaxants, 80, 174
Myelogram, 16

N

National Institute of Occupational Safety and
    Health, 148, 149
Nelson bed, 84, 90, 93
Nerve root irritation syndrome, 17, 175
Nesacaine; *see* Chloroprocaine
Neurological compression, 2
Neurological deficit, 42
Neuroprobe, 84
NIOSH; *see* National Institute of Occupational
    Safety and Health
Nucleus pulposus, herniated, 28, 29, 32, *33,*
    34
Nutrition, 179

O

Object factor guidelines, 148
Obstacle course, 15, 49-52
  general, testing, 53-64
Operant conditioning program, 81

Operators
   equipment, reducing back stress in, 155-156
   seated and standing, 152-154
Osteophyte formation, 32

P

Pain, 179; *see also* Symptoms, athletics and
    severity of
   aggravated by sitting and flexing, 40
   back, 40; *see also* Low back pain
    acute, 39t, 175
    chronic, 176
   back and leg
    acute, 41t
    chronic, 41t
   buttock, 40
   from extension and rotation, 40
   graph for recording, after injections, *18*
   leg, 40
   low back; *see* Low back pain
Pain drawing, *12,* 13
Pain history, 4
Pain rehabilitation inpatient program, 94-95
Pain scale, *13,* 14
Palpation, 14, 15
Patient
   evaluation of
    etiology of low back pain and, 1-25
    summary of, 25
    working, 74-76
   handling of; *see* Patient handling
Patient handling, 97-106
   gurney transfers, 102-103
   in bed, 98-99
   and lifting problems, 103-106
   pushing and pulling, 99
   wheelchair transfers, 101-102
Patient instruction, basic back school, 66, 72-
    74
PCI; *see* Personal Concerns Inventory
Pelvic tilt, *67,* 72, 117
Pentothal; *see* Thiopental
Personal Concerns Inventory, 10-11
Physical condition guidelines, employee, 150
Physical examination, 15-16; *see also* Eval-
    uation, physical
Pool therapy, 176
Position(s)
   awkward, 130-131
   knee-chest, 15
   lying, proper, 107

Position(s)—cont'd
   neutral, 90
   seated; *see* Sitting
   standing; *see* Standing
Posture, abnormalities in, 14
Preemployment selection, 150
Prevention of back injuries, 143-144
Program(s)
   athletic training, 162-164
   general fitness, in industry, 144
   safety, industrial, 147
Psychological diagnosis, 28-29t
Psychological environment, 80-81
Psychological low back pain, 38-39
Psychological testing, 4
Psychologists, 140
Pushing and pulling in industry, 151-152
Pushup, partial, 15

R

Raney flexion body jacket, 173
Reaching and climbing, 132
Reinforcement for employees, 144
Relaxants, muscle, 80, 174
Relaxation therapy, 80
Responsibility, 143
Rest periods, 138
Ricarro seat, 116
Running and jogging, 164-166

S

Safety program in industry, 147
Safeway Stores, Inc., 46, 142, 144
Schedules, basic back school, 50, 70-71, 77, 78
School(s)
   back; *see* Back school
   future of back school in, 177-178
Sclerosing agents, 176
Scoliosis, 28-29t
   and postural strain, 35-36
Seat, Ricarro, 116
Seat belts, use of, 155
Seated position; *see* Sitting
Self-mobilization, 84, 171
Sex, 132-133
Shoe lifts, 176
Shoes, 137
Shower, taking, 133-134
Sitting, 112-117, 129; *see also* Operators,
    seated and standing
   on ground, 114-115

Sitting—cont'd
for long periods, 116-117
in motor vehicles, 115-116
proper position for, 112
in straight back chairs, 114
Sit-up, partial, 74, *75*, 126
Skier's position, 74, *75*, 127
Snook, Stover, 147-148, 177
Soccer, 160
Social and emotional factors, employee,
150
Social Readjustment Rating Scale, 6
Social workers, 140
Southern Pacific Transportation Companies, 46,
142, 146
Spasms, 49
Spinal insufficiency, 26
Spinal stenosis, 28-29t, 36-37, 84
Spondylitis, ankylosing, 28-29t, 36
Spondylolisthesis, 28-29t, 35, 84
Spondylolysis, 34
Sports; *see* Back school, athletic
Sports medicine center, 79
Sprain
back, 37-38
soft tissue, 38
SRRS; *see* Social Readjustment Rating
Scale
Standing
and walking at home, 117
at work, 152, 154
Statistics, back school, 45-47
successful, 46t
Stenosis, spinal, 28-29t, 36-37, 84
Steroids, 24
Straight backbend, 72, 124
Straight leg raising, 15, 23, 42, 49, *89*
Strain, scoliosis and postural, 35-36
Stress, 139
heat, and other environmental considerations,
149-150
postural, minimizing, in truck drivers,
155
Stress management, 133
Surgery, selection for, 169-170
Surgical hospital program, before and after,
93-94
Swedish low back school, 44
Swimming, 158
Symptoms, athletics and severity of, 157-158
moderately disabled and painful, 158

Symptoms—cont'd
severe pain and disability, 157
Syndrome
facet, 17
arthritis, 175
nerve root irritation, 17, 175

T

Technique factor guidelines, 148
Tennis, 158, 159, 166, *167*
Tension, 174-175
emotional, 139
Testing
general obstacle course, 53-64
psychological, 4
Tests
air acceptance, 19
diagnostic, 16-18, 93
exercise tolerance, 76
Faber, 15
flip, 15
hanging drop, 19
Hendler 10-Minute Screening, 7-9
Hoover, 15
Lasegue, 15
Therapists
occupational, 140
physical, 44-45, 93, 140
as patient managers, 94
Therapy, 42
recommended, low back pain patients,
28-29t
relaxation, 80
Thiopental, 24
Tilt table, 90, 93
Toilets
arrangement of, 136
sitting on, 118, *119*
Tomography, 16-17
Traction, 84, 179
gravity lumbar, 174
inverted gravity, 84
Transcutaneous stimulation, postoperative, 93
Transcutaneous stimulators, 84
Treatment
conservative, 169-176
extension, 40
flexion, 40

U

Ultrasound, 176

V

Vacuum cleaner, selecting, 135
Vacuuming, 127-128
Venogram, epidural, 16, 17
Vertebra chair, 116
Vibration effects, minimizing, in truck drivers, 155
Vitamins, 176

W

Walking and standing, 117
Wall slide, 74, *75,* 127
Waterbeds, 107
Weight lifting, 158, *159*
Wood, chopping, 129
Work
    and environment design guidelines, 146-156
    height of, 149

Work—cont'd
    around house, 127-129
    return to, 117
Work environment; *see* Back school in the work environment
Work load, 149
Work space
    sitting, 153
    standing, 154
Work surface, height and inclination of
    for sitting position, 153
    for standing position, 154
Working patient, 74-76

X

X-ray films, 16
Xylocaine; *see* Lidocaine